*Barry N. Checkoway, PhD*
*Lorraine M. Gutiérrez, PhD*
*Editors*

# Youth Participation
# and Community Change

*Youth Participation and Community Change* has been
co-published simultaneously as *Journal of Community Practice*, Volume 14, Numbers 1/2 2006.

*Pre-publication*
*REVIEWS,*
*COMMENTARIES,*
*EVALUATIONS . . .*

"**R**EFRESHING AND EXCITING. . . .
An INFORMATIVE AND THOU-
GHT-PROVOKING volume that
should be read by community organizers, youth workers, and advocates."

**Michael S. Reisch, PhD, MSW**
*Professor*
*School of Social Work*
*University of Michigan*

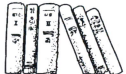

D0224622

The Haworth Press, Inc.

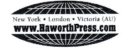

New York • London • Victoria (AU)
**www.HaworthPress.com**

# Youth Participation
# and Community Change

*Youth Participation and Community Change* has been co-published simultaneously as *Journal of Community Practice*, Volume 14, Numbers 1/2 2006.

Randolph,
with best wishes!
Barry

# Monographic Separates from the *Journal of Community Practice*™

For additional information on these and other Haworth Press titles, including descriptions, tables of contents, reviews, and prices, use the QuickSearch catalog at http://www.HaworthPress.com.

*Youth Participation and Community Change,* edited by Barry N. Checkoway, PhD, and Lorraine M. Gutiérrez, PhD (Vol. 14, No. 1/2, 2006). *"REFRESHING AND EXCITING . . . . An INFORMATIVE AND THOUGHT-PROVOKING volume that should be read by community organizers, youth workers, and advocates." (Michael S. Reisch, PhD, MSW, Professor, School of Social Work, University of Michigan)*

*University-Community Partnerships: Universities in Civic Engagement,* edited by Tracy M. Soska, MSW, and Alice K. Johnson Butterfield, PhD (Vol. 12, No. 3/4, 2004). *Community Outreach Partnership Centers (COPC), sponsored by the United States Department of Housing and Urban Development (HUD), have identified civic engagement and community partnership as critical themes for higher education. This unique book addresses past, present, and future models of university-community partnerships, COPC programs, wide-ranging social work partnerships that involve teaching research, and social change, and innovative methods in the processes of civic engagement.*

*Innovative Approaches for Teaching Community Organization Skills in the Classroom,* edited by Donna Hardina, PhD (Vol. 7, No. 1, 2000). *This accessible and comprehensive book will help social work educators efficiently teach students methods of practice that they need to know in order to offer the best services to clients with a variety of different needs, in a variety of different settings.*

*Research Strategies for Community Practice,* edited by Ray H. MacNair, PhD, MSW (Supp. #1, 1998). *"An excellent compilation of materials. A key sourcebook for ideas on community organization research." (John Tropman, PhD, Professor, School of Social Work, University of Michigan, Ann Arbor)*

*Community Economic Development and Social Work,* edited by Margaret S. Sherraden, PhD, and William A. Ninacs, MS, CED (Vol. 5, No. 1/2, 1998). *"The major value of this book is its potential to bring together the two opposing streams of thinking about social welfare. Both liberals and conservatives can rally around the approach explicated in this book." (Roland Meiner, PhD, President, Missouri Association for Social Welfare)*

*Community Practice: Models in Action,* edited by Marie Weil, DSW (Vol. 4, No. 1, 1997). *"The text stands alone among macro tests in its timeliness, comprehensiveness, and contribution to strategy development–it could well become a classic." (Moses Newsome, Jr., PhD, Dean, School of Social Work, Norfolk State University; President, Council on Social Work Education)*

*Community Practice: Conceptual Models,* edited by Marie Weil, DSW (Vol. 3, No. 3/4, 1996). *"Presents diverse views on approaches to community practice and provides a compilation, critique, and analysis of current models while illustrating how these approaches have developed over time." (Public Welfare)*

*African American Community Practice Models: Historical and Contemporary Responses,* edited by Iris Carlton-LaNey, PhD, and N. Yolanda Burwell, PhD (Vol. 2, No. 4, 1996). *"If you're a social worker who cares about today's and tomorrow's African American communities, read this book. . . . It's likely to become a classic in its own right." (Paul H. Ephross, PhD, Professor, School of Social Work, University of Maryland at Baltimore)*

*Diversity and Development in Community Practice,* edited by Audrey Faulkner, PhD, Maria Roberts-DeGennaro, PhD, and Marie Weil, DSW (Vol. 1, No. 1, 1993). *The contributing authors provide current knowledge and practice models for community work in diverse settings.*

# Youth Participation and Community Change

Barry N. Checkoway, PhD
Lorraine M. Gutiérrez, PhD
Editors

*Youth Participation and Community Change* has been co-published simultaneously as *Journal of Community Practice*, Volume 14, Numbers 1/2 2006.

The Haworth Press, Inc.

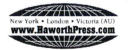

New York • London • Victoria (AU)
www.HaworthPress.com

*Youth Participation and Community Change* has been co-published simultaneously as *Journal of Community Practice*™, Volume 14, Numbers 1/2 2006.

The development, preparation, and publication of this work has been undertaken with great care. However, the publisher, employees, editors, and agents of The Haworth Press and all imprints of The Haworth Press, Inc., including The Haworth Medical Press® and Pharmaceutical Products Press®, are not responsible for any errors contained herein or for consequences that may ensue from use of materials or information contained in this work.

The Haworth Press is commited to the dissemination of ideas and information according to the highest standards of intellectual freedom and the free exchange of ideas. Statements made and opinions expressed in this publication do not necessarily reflect the views of the Publisher, Directors, management, or staff of The Haworth Press, Inc., or an endorsement by them.

Cover design by Jennifer Gaska

Cover Photo: The photograph on the cover was taken by Naomi Milstein. The group represents Youth Dialogues on Race and Ethnicity in Metropolitan Detroit, a program made possible with support from the Skillman Foundation and University of Michigan.

**Library of Congress Cataloging-in-Publication Data**

Checkoway, Barry.
    Youth Participation and Community Change / Barry N. Checkoway, Lorraine M. Gutiérrez, editors.
        p. cm.
        "Youth Participation and Community Change has been co-published simultaneously as Journal of Community Practice, Volume 14, Numbers 1/2, 2006."
        Includes bibliographical references and index.
        ISBN 13: 978-0-7890-3291-1 (hard cover : alk. paper)
        ISBN 10: 0-7890-3291-0 (hard cover: alk. paper)
        ISBN 13: 978-0-7890-3292-8 (soft cover : alk.paper)
        ISBN 10: 0-7890-3292-9 (soft cover : alk.paper)
        1. Young volunteers in community development. 2. Young volunteers. 3. Leadership. 4. Community development. I. Gutiérrez, Lorraine M. (Lorraine Margot). II. Journal of Community Practice. III. Title.
    HN90.V64C485 2006
    307.1′40835–dc22                                                                2006000952

# Indexing, Abstracting & Website/Internet Coverage

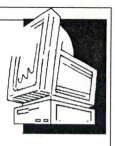

This section provides you with a list of major indexing & abstracting services and other tools for bibliographic access. That is to say, each service began covering this periodical during the year noted in the right column. Most Websites which are listed below have indicated that they will either post, disseminate, compile, archive, cite or alert their own Website users with research-based content from this work. (This list is as current as the copyright date of this publication.)

Abstracting, Website/Indexing Coverage . . . . . . . . Year When Coverage Began

- *Alternative Press Index (print, online & CD-ROM from NISC)*
  *The most complete guide to alternative & radical media*
  *<http://www.altpress.org>* . . . . . . . . . . . . . . . . . . . . . . . . . . . . . . **1995**
- *Applied Social Sciences Index & Abstracts (ASSIA)*
  *(Online: ASSI via DataStar) (CDRom: ASSIA Plus)*
  *<http://www.csa.com>* . . . . . . . . . . . . . . . . . . . . . . . . . . . . . . . **1994**
- *Business Source Corporate: coverage of nearly 3,350 quality*
  *magazines and journals; designed to meet the diverse information*
  *needs of corporations; EBSCO Publishing*
  *<http://www.epnet.com/corporate/bsourcecorp.asp>* . . . . . . . . . . **2002**
- *CareData: the database supporting social care management*
  *and practice <http://www.elsc.org.uk/caredata/caredata.htm>* . . . **1994**
- *CINAHL (Cumulative Index to Nursing & Allied Health*
  *Literature), in print, EBSCO, and SilverPlatter, DataStar,*
  *and PaperChase (Support materials include Subject Heading*
  *List, Database Search Guide, and instructional video)*
  *<http://www.cinahl.com>* . . . . . . . . . . . . . . . . . . . . . . . . . . . . . . **1996**
- *EBSCOhost Electronic Journals Service (EJS)*
  *<http://ejournals.ebsco.com>* . . . . . . . . . . . . . . . . . . . . . . . . . . . **2001**
- *Elsevier Scopus <http://www.info.scopus.com>* . . . . . . . . . . . . . . . **2005**
- *Environmental Sciences and Pollution Management (Cambridge*
  *Scientific Abstracts Internet Database Service)*
  *<http://www.csa.com>* . . . . . . . . . . . . . . . . . . . . . . . . . . . . . . . **2003**
- *Family & Society Studies Worldwide <http://www.nisc.com>* . . . . . . **1995**

(continued)

(continued)

*Special bibliographic notes related to special journal issues (separates) and indexing/abstracting:*

- indexing/abstracting services in this list will also cover material in any "separate" that is co-published simultaneously with Haworth's special thematic journal issue or DocuSerial. Indexing/abstracting usually covers material at the article/chapter level.
- monographic co-editions are intended for either non-subscribers or libraries which intend to purchase a second copy for their circulating collections.
- monographic co-editions are reported to all jobbers/wholesalers/approval plans. The source journal is listed as the "series" to assist the prevention of duplicate purchasing in the same manner utilized for books-in-series.
- to facilitate user/access services all indexing/abstracting services are encouraged to utilize the co-indexing entry note indicated at the bottom of the first page of each article/chapter/contribution.
- this is intended to assist a library user of any reference tool (whether print, electronic, online, or CD-ROM) to locate the monographic version if the library has purchased this version but not a subscription to the source journal.
- individual articles/chapters in any Haworth publication are also available through the Haworth Document Delivery Service (HDDS).

# Youth Participation and Community Change

## CONTENTS

## YOUTH PARTICIPATION IN EVALUATION AND RESEARCH

## STUDENT FACILITATORS AND COLLABORATIVE TEAMS FOR PARTICIPATION

# ABOUT THE EDITORS

**Barry Checkoway, PhD, MA,** is Professor of Social Work and Urban Planning, and Founding Director of the Ginsberg Center for Community Service and Learning at the University of Michigan, where he teaches courses in community organization, community planning, and community development. He has extensive experience in working with grassroots groups to participate in community institutions that affect their lives, and with community agencies to involve community representatives in their decisions. These include work with groups in the South Bronx, Detroit, Mississippi Delta, Albuquerque, Oakland, and other areas. Professor Checkoway's publications include books and articles for professional and popular audiences in the fields of social work, urban planning, public health, youth development, community participation, and program evaluation. His publications include *Youth Participation in Community Planning* (with Ramona Mullahey and Yve Susskind), *Young People Creating Community Change*, and *Participatory Evaluation with Young People* (with Katie Richards-Schuster).

**Lorraine M. Gutiérrez, PhD, MA,** is an internationally recognized scholar in the area of multicultural theory and practice. She has published more than 35 books, chapters, and articles on topics such as multicultural organizational and community development, working with women of color, group work, empowerment practice, and community-based research. She teaches courses in multicultural practice, action research, and community work in the Department of Psychology and School of Social Work at the University of Michigan, and currently directs the Joint Interdisciplinary Doctoral Program in Social Work and Social Science. In addition to her scholarship and teaching, Dr. Gutiérrez provides consultation to large and small organizations. This includes faculty development workshops at the annual meetings of the Council on Social Work Education, work with the Swedish National Board of Health and Welfare, and consultation with social work schools throughout the United States. She has a strong commitment to using her scholarship to benefit neighborhoods and communities.

# Youth Participation and Community Change: An Introduction

Barry N. Checkoway, PhD
Lorraine M. Gutiérrez, PhD

Youth participation is a process of involving young people in the institutions and decisions that affect their lives. It includes initiatives that emphasize educational reform, juvenile justice, environmental quality, and other issues; that involve populations distinguished by class, race, gender, and other characteristics; and that operate in rural areas, small towns, suburbs, and neighborhoods of large cities in developing areas and industrial nations worldwide.

As expressions of participation, young people are organizing groups for social and political action, planning programs of their own choosing, and advocating their interests in the community. They are raising consciousness, educating others on matters that concern them, and providing services of their own choosing. No single strategy characterizes all approaches to participation.

Activities like these can be conceptualized in various ways. For example, Roger Hart (1997) identifies activities and places them on the rungs of a vertical "ladder of participation" in accordance with the power they exercise; Danny HoSang (2003) analyzes youth organizing, youth development, and other models on a horizontal continuum; and

[Haworth co-indexing entry note]: "Youth Participation and Community Change: An Introduction." Checkoway, Barry N., and Lorraine M. Gutiérrez. Co-published simultaneously in *Journal of Community Practice* (The Haworth Press, Inc.) Vol. 14, No. 1/2, 2006, pp. 1-9; and: *Youth Participation and Community Change* (ed: Barry N. Checkoway, and Lorraine M. Gutiérrez) The Haworth Press, Inc., 2006, pp. 1-9. Single or multiple copies of this article are available for a fee from The Haworth Document Delivery Service [1-800-HAWORTH, 9:00 a.m. - 5:00 p.m. (EST). E-mail address: docdelivery@haworthpress.com].

*1*

David Driskell (2002) describes several "steps in the process" from gathering information to program evaluation.

These activities have potential to produce outcomes at multiple levels. Studies of several population groups show that participation can strengthen social development, build organizational capacity, and create changes in the environment. There has been relatively little systematic study of youth participation outcomes at multiple levels, but the research with other populations suggests that studies with youth will find positive effects on such measures as personal confidence, social connectedness, civic competencies, and leadership development. At present, however, the potential benefits of participation on youth have not been identified by systematic research.

Youth participation is about the real influence of young people in institutions and decisions, not about their passive presence as human subjects or service recipients. Although participation studies often assess activities in terms of their scope–such as their number, frequency, and duration–quality is their most significant measure. Just because a number of young people attend a number of meetings and speak a number of times, is no measure of their effect. Quality participation shows some effect on outcomes, including its effect on community change.

Youth participation includes efforts by young people to plan programs of their own choosing; by adults to involve young people in their agencies; and by youth and adults to work together in intergenerational partnerships. However, the issue is not whether the effort is youth-led, adult-led, or intergenerational, but rather whether young people have actual effect.

Youth participation is consistent with the view of "youth as resources," and contrasts with the image of "youth as problems" that permeates the popular media, social science, and professional practice when referring to young people.

For example, the media often portray young people, especially young people of color, as perpetrators of crime, drug takers, school dropouts, or other problems of society. With these images in mind, many adults think of young people as problems, and young people accept adult images of their deficiencies rather than viewing themselves as agents of change.

Social scientists reinforce this view with studies of poverty, racism, and other forces that cause poor housing, broken families, and worsening social conditions, and result in youth violence, drug abuse, and other social pathologies that require intervention.

Social workers and other professionals who adopt this view of young people seek to save, protect, and defend them from conditions that affect them. When the curricula at professional schools construct youth as victims of society, professionals are prepared roles in helping them and their families do something about their terrible personal and social conditions. When people focus on others' needs and deficiencies, it de-emphasizes their assets and strengths, weakens their ability to help themselves, and empowers the professionals who serve them.

However, another view that portrays young people as competent citizens with a right to participate and a responsibility to serve their communities provides a significant alternative. Proponents of this view want to build on the strengths of youth by enabling them to make a difference in ways that provide them with tangible benefits and develop healthier communities. Young people who view themselves as change agents, and adults who are their allies, are instrumental to this approach.

Social workers are strategically situated to promote youth participation, but many of them have been conditioned to "care" about young people rather than to "empower" them. Those social workers who emphasize the rights of young people to participate in society and their responsibilities to serve the community are not typical of the field.

There are explanations for why this might be the case. For example, Janet Finn (2001) argues that social workers are agents of an "adolescent pathology industry" which provides services to "troubled and troubling" young and perpetuates their roles as passive recipients rather than active participants. Whatever the explanation, social workers still have substantial contact with young people which offers opportunities for them to promote active participation rather than provide reactive services.

Youth participation can be expected to increase in the future. Several private foundations have increased their funding for community organizations and civic agencies; national associations have expanded their support for local initiatives; and intermediary organizations have broadened their training and technical assistance. Recent conferences and publications have increased awareness among popular and professional audiences, and there is talk of a "youth participation movement" in the making.

More knowledge of youth participation as a subject of study will contribute to its quality as a field of practice. We surmise that participation has several strategies, that their activities have effects at multiple levels, and that their outcomes are influenced by forces that facilitate or limit them. However, we know that there is too little systematic research, and that more knowledge of participation will strengthen their practice.

This volume provides new perspectives on youth participation in organizations and communities. It considers the changing context of youth participation, models and methods of participatory practice, roles of youth and adults, and the future of youth and community in a diverse democracy. It includes approaches which promote participatory community-based research and evaluation, and involve youth groups in economically dis-invested and racially segregated areas.

The articles in this collection are diverse, including conceptual and theoretical discussions, empirically-based case studies and best practices, and interdisciplinary work that draws upon psychology, sociology, social work, public health, education, and related academic disciplines and professional fields. The authors include youth and adult practitioners, researchers, and educators whose experience and expertise are not always represented in publications like this.

The first articles provide conceptual frameworks for understanding young people and their participation. In contrast to "youth as problems," Silvia Blitzer Golombeck defines "youth as citizens," a concept consistent with the United Nations Convention on the Rights of the Child. Rather than emphasizing the age of young people as a defining characteristic of citizenship, she emphasizes their involvement in civic activities. She offers examples from a Norwegian city whose strategic plan identifies young people as "fellow citizens" and from an American city whose youth participate in the urban planning process, as a way to substantiate her definition.

Louise B. Jennings, Deborah M. Parra-Medina, DeAnne K. Hilfinger Messias, and Kerry McLoughlin formulate a critical social theory of youth empowerment as a way to understand youth participation. They draw upon a number of existing empowerment models–including adolescent empowerment, youth development, transactional partnering, and the empowerment education model formulated by Paulo Friere–as a basis for framing their own notion of participation whose dimensions include assessing its effects at the individual and community levels.

What are some ways to prepare young people for active participation in a diverse democracy? Esminia M. Luluquisen, and Alma M. O. Trinidad, and Dipankar Ghosh describe Hawaii's *Sariling Gawa* youth council as an approach to youth leadership which is consistent with empowerment principles and which promotes positive ethnic social identity, and builds organizational and community capacity, of Filipino youth. Through this program, young people set priorities, formulate plans, and organize action groups. They attend cultural events, conduct community conferences, and complete service projects. In the face of discrimination, they position themselves for social change.

Melanie D. Otis describes the Lexington Youth Leadership Academy as an effort to prepare participants for leadership roles. Young people develop knowledge for problem solving, program planning, peer mentoring, and community collaboration through a program which includes dialogues on diversity and a community change agent project. Program evaluators assess its effects on their self-concept, social action orientation, and other measures.

Cindy Carlson describes an exemplary effort in Hampton, Virginia to engage young people in public policy at the municipal level. Starting with a city council decision to create a coalition and make the city a better place for youth, they have developed a multi-tiered system of participation opportunities, including a youth commission which involves young people in public policy and leadership development. As part of the process, they address attitudes and create cultural changes among adults that fail to recognize young people as resources. She shows that the municipality has real potential for youth participation, and identifies "adults as allies" in addition to youth leaders as key participants.

Participatory research and evaluation are ways to involve young people in community change. In contrast to the usual pattern in which knowledge development is viewed as a process in which technical experts conduct research and ordinary people play passive roles, participatory research is an approach in which people collaborate in defining problems, gathering information, analyzing findings, and using the knowledge. Although this approach is increasing among adult groups distinguished by class, race, gender, and other characteristics, young people are not normally at the table.

Our authors have a different take. For example, Kysa Nygreen, Soo Ah Kwon, and Patricia Sánchez assume that young people can and should participate in the research process, and report on efforts to involve three different groups of urban youth who are normally marginalized, namely a multi-ethnic school-based group of students transforming curriculum in an alternative high school, a Latina group conducting research on transnational experiences, and pan-ethnic Asian and Pacific Island groups focused on youth organizing and social justice. They conclude that these youth are a vital resource for community transformation.

Ahna Ballonoff Suleiman, Samira Soleimanpour, and Jonathan London examine efforts by young people to participate in research projects in seven school-based health centers. The notion that the schools are a vehicle for using research as a form of education for democracy is not new, but the promise of this approach is generally not realized. The authors describe specific strategies and reflect on the lessons learned from these initiatives.

Caroline C. Wang describes photovoice as a particular participatory action research tool for involving young people in communities. She describes an approach in which youth employ cameras to record their community's strengths and concerns, promote critical dialogue about community issues through group discussion of photographs, and communicate their concerns to policy makers. She draws upon data from ten projects in which youth used photovoice to advocate community health and well-being.

Youth participation in research and evaluation is an international movement, which is also represented by our authors. For example, Reima Ana Maglajlić, Jennifer Tiffany, and their colleagues describe participatory research in Bosnia and Herzegovina, an area affected by political violence in recent years. With support from a global UNICEF initiative, adults launched a project in which young people in three towns assessed conditions related to HIV/AIDS, drug use, and human rights. Young researchers gathered information and produced recommendations.

Louise Chawla and David Driskell describe the Growing Up in Cities Project supported by UNESCO, an initiative inspired by the United Nations Convention on the Rights of the Child to promote participation in communities. They describe a case study in Bangalore, India in which young people played active roles. They conclude that young people are able and willing to participate in this way, that the most effective approach is when youth and adults work together, and that adult decision makers do not always have accurate information about such possibilities.

Who has responsibility for facilitation of youth participation? Although participation initiatives might be youth-led, adult-led, or intergenerational in their origins, we recognize that none of the ones described here is truly youth-led. However, we reiterate that the quality of participation is not contingent on this approach, and that it is as likely that quality youth participation might be adult-led or intergenerational as it is that youth leadership might not be participatory.

Some authors address the roles of young people as peer facilitators. Nance Wilson, Meredith Minkler, Stefan Dasho, Roxanne Carrillo, Nina Wallerstein, and Diego Garcia describe the training of high school and graduate students as peer facilitators of a university-community partnership which involves elementary school students in research which promotes problem-solving, social action, and civic participation among underserved elementary school youth. Their work represents a youth-to-youth model in which some young people learn best from others who are slightly older and have more experience than they.

Julie A. Scheve, Daniel F. Perkins, and Claudia Mincemoyer describe collaborative teams in which youth and adults work together in intergenerational partnerships. Because young people are often isolated from adults, this approach enables them to connect with adult allies, gain adult support, and collaborate in activities which have potential for community change.

Youth development or youth organizing? Although social workers often conceptualize youth participation as a form of youth development and distinguish this from traditional provision of services to at-risk youth, young people also play roles as organizers and planners of initiatives which increase their involvement and build healthier communities.

None of the articles here is about youth organizing as an approach in which young people take initiative and organize groups on their own. Michelle Alberti Gambone, Hanh Cao Yu, Heather Lewis-Charp, Cynthia L. Sipe, and Johanna Lacoe examine the differences among these and other efforts. They examine different types of agencies and find that there are significant differences in outcomes among youth organizing, identity-support, and traditional youth development organizations in terms of outcomes like civic activism and identity development. Youth organizing agencies show higher levels of youth leadership, decision making, and community involvement. There is no a priori reason why youth development efforts cannot serve as a vehicle for activism, but their research suggests that this is not now the case.

Overall, we are heartened that social workers, public health workers, and others are increasing the involvement of young people in the community, reflecting upon their experience, and writing about the lessons learned from empirically-based practice. We believe that strengthening youth participation as a subject study will contribute to the scope and quality of its practice, and hope that these articles will contribute to the process.

Social workers and other professionals are ideally positioned for strengthening youth participation for community change. If only a fraction of them were to take leadership for fostering this work in their respective fields, the results would be significant.

It is a pleasure to acknowledge some of those whose work made this volume possible. We appreciate the editors of the *Journal of Community Practice* for their encouragement of our efforts, Katie Richards-Schuster for her experience and expertise with the content of the work, and Ana Santiago for her management of the process from the initial call for papers to the final preparation of manuscripts. We also appreciate our many reviewers, for their collegial contributions to our common purpose.

## REFERENCES

Driskell, D. (2002). *Creating better cities with children and youth: A manual for participation*. Paris/London: Earthscan/Unesco Publishing.

Finn, J.L. (2001). Text and turbulence: Representing adolescence as pathology in the human services. *Childhood, 8*, 167-192.

Hart, R.D. (1997). *Children's participation: The theory and practice of involving young citizens in community development and environmental care*. New York/London: Unicef/Earthscan.

HoSang, D. (2003). *Youth and community organizing today*. New York: Funders' Collaborative on Youth Organizing.

## *LIST OF SPECIAL ISSUE REVIEWERS: YOUTH PARTICIPATION AND COMMUNITY CHANGE*

A special thanks to those who reviewed for this collection, including:

Terrence Allen, Ann Rosegrant Alvarez, Tony Alvarez, Darlyne Bailey, Rick Battistoni, Adam Becker, Marcia Bombyk, Gary L. Bowen, Pam Brown, Julio Cammarota, E. Summerson Carr, Louise Chawla, Julian Chow, Melvin Delgado, Dave Dobbie, Jacquelynne Eccles, Kristin Michelle Ferguson, Janet Finn, Robert Fisher, Connie Flanagan, Sondra Fogel, Helen Fox, Andy Furco, Dee Gamble, Larry Gant, Charles Garvin, Dwight Giles, Shawn Ginwright, Leslie Goodyear, Lorraine Gutiérrez, Yael Harlap, Danny HoSang, Jeff Howard, Cheryl Hyde, Merita Irby, Jane Isaacs-Lowe, Francine Jacobs, Alice Johnson Butterfield, Debra Jozefowicz-Simbeni, Michele A. Kelley, Richard Lerner, Jonathan London, Flavio Marsiglia, Bart Miles, A. T. Miller, Meredith Minkler, David P. Moxley, Ramona Mullahey, Elizabeth Mulroy, Susan Murty, Ann Weaver Nichols, Phil Nyden, Yolanda

Padilla, S. Mark Pancer, Edith Parker, Kameshwari Pothukuchi, Michael Reisch, Cynthia Rocha, Kim Sabo, Izumi Sakamoto, Ramón Salcido, Rosemary Sarri, Jean Schensul, Margaret Sherrard-Sherraden, Carmen Sirianni, Lee Staples, Swojciech Sokolowski, Tracy Soska, Teri Sullivan, Yve Susskind, Martin B. Tracy, Diane Vinokur, Alicia Wilson-Ahlstrom, Nina Wallerstein, Karen Young, Nicole Yohalem, and Richard Shep Zeldin.

# Children as Citizens

## Silvia Blitzer Golombek, PhD

**SUMMARY.** This article makes the case for a definition of citizenship that emphasizes the civic participation activities of young people rather than an age at which they receive formal recognition as citizens. It provides a conceptual framework and some of the arguments which favor a definition of this type, and draws upon examples from the youth service, service-learning, and youth in decision-making fields from the United States and other countries, which support the notion that children are not "citizens in the making" but instead social agents who already participate in building strong and democratic communities. *[Article copies available for a fee from The Haworth Document Delivery Service: 1-800-HAWORTH. E-mail address: <docdelivery@haworthpress.com> Website: <http://www.HaworthPress.com> © 2006 by The Haworth Press, Inc. All rights reserved.]*

**KEYWORDS.** Citizenship, civic participation, international, service-learning, volunteering, young children

Silvia Blitzer Golombek is Vice President of Programs, Youth Service America (E-mail: sgolombek@ysa.org).

[Haworth co-indexing entry note]: "Children as Citizens." Golombek, Silvia Blitzer. Co-published simultaneously in *Journal of Community Practice* (The Haworth Press, Inc.) Vol. 14, No. 1/2, 2006, pp. 11-30; and: *Youth Participation and Community Change* (ed: Barry N. Checkoway, and Lorraine M. Gutiérrez) The Haworth Press, Inc., 2006, pp. 11-30. Single or multiple copies of this article are available for a fee from The Haworth Document Delivery Service [1-800-HAWORTH, 9:00 a.m. - 5:00 p.m. (EST). E-mail address: docdelivery@haworthpress.com].

doi:10.1300/J125v14n01_02

## INTRODUCTION

Who is a citizen? Common definitions refer to individuals who have been born in a particular country ("jus solis"), are children of parents born in that country ("jus sanguinis") or become citizens of a nation by choice. In the United States the concept also is associated to a person's change in status at the age of 18 by which he or she acquires the right to vote in elections for public office along with other rights and responsibilities, including full employment, entering into contracts, and marriage. Citizenship, therefore, is understood as an affiliation with a nation-state and as a series of duties and rights acquired because of age. These definitions, however, leave out other behaviors that, if taken into account, broaden the concept of citizenship to include other activities that engage individuals in public life. By that expanded definition, children and youth under 18 can be considered citizens as well, regardless of place of birth.

The discussion that follows seeks to make the case for an expanded definition of citizenship that focuses on certain *activities* undertaken by individuals rather than on the parameters of *age* and *status* when those individuals are actually recognized as citizens. The article will focus primarily on different streams of community service activities as a key skill and responsibility of "citizenship." The following sections present first a conceptual framework to understand some of the dimensions inherent to commonly used definitions of citizenship and possible arguments to expand that definition to view younger children's activities through a citizenship lens. This is followed by a brief description of two cases–one in Norway and one in the United States–that incorporate children as citizens in innovative ways. Next, a review of program examples and cases drawn from the youth service, service learning, and youth participation fields both in the United States and in other countries show children's active engagement in community improvement and social change and support an expanded definition of citizenship that includes minors. The paper concludes with the discussion of some of the barriers, implications, and opportunities associated with the consideration of younger children as citizens.

## WHAT IS CITIZENSHIP?

"Citizenship is the social and legal link between individuals and their democratic political community" (Patrick, 2000, p. 5). It is commonly defined as a legal status with duties such as paying taxes, serving in the armed forces, obeying the laws, and participating in community improvement efforts. Citizens also enjoy certain rights such as voting, participating in public interest groups, and being elected for public office. While in the United States of America only citizens can vote in general elections, serve on juries, and be elected to certain offices, everyone–including noncitizens–enjoy all other rights.

As defined above, activities such as writing letters to local newspapers to express opinions about a community issue, organizing a neighborhood clean up project, meeting with public officials to request the placement of stop signs at dangerous street intersections, participating in interest groups and organizations, or publicly debating the proposed building of a ten-story garage to replace a historical landmark are expressions of citizenship. In each of these instances, individuals engage in activities that connect them to larger issues to sustain and strengthen their community–the traits of "good citizens."

It is clear that adults engage and are expected to participate in these behaviors. However, adults are not the only ones involved in such activities on a daily basis; so are children under 18 although conventional definitions of citizenship do not include minors as active participants in community building. As the examples presented later in this article confirm, children are engaging in civic activities: voting for school governments and town budgets, advocating for policy changes, and conducting multiple activities "to improve the quality of political and civic life" (Patrick, 2000, p. 6), although their activities are often considered only learning experiences or preparation for responsible citizenship as adults.

The notion of citizenship, therefore, is dynamic and multidimensional: from a legal standpoint, it defines rights and responsibilities restricted only to those born in a particular country and have reached a certain age to fulfill certain tasks like voting for elected officials or serving in the military. In different countries or historical periods, citizens' rights and duties have been and still are restricted by gender and ethnicity as well. However, while minors do not vote in general elections in the United States, they (native and immigrant) do engage in "political" activity when voting for school government and youth councils; they also must abide by the laws (although sanctions for their infringement are qualified by age). And behaviors like donating money and time to social causes reflect other key dimensions of citizenship directed at building and strengthening community.

Marc Jans (2004) reflects on these different dimensions and questions whether it is meaningful to apply an adult-centric notion of citizenship to children and in what way can children be seen as citizens. He argues that if citizenship is defined as "whole rights" (voting for public officials), the definition applies only to adults. A definition of citizenship as a set of responsibilities (being responsible and following the rules), does not take into account that children change game rules and do not fulfill certain responsibilities, for example, without severe consequences. Defining citizenship as an identity only applies to children when referring to an immediate environment and varies with maturity level: young children feel a sense of belonging to a family or their school class, but have not necessarily internalized their identity as Italian, European or Latin American. "Because of the progressive way in which children appropriate their environment, at first mainly local forms of citizenship are within the reach of children" (p. 39). It is a definition of citizenship as participation ("I feel involved and can participate in community life") that seems to apply to children with fewer limitations. The cases of children's participation described in this article are a few of the numerous ways in which children are expressing their sense of belonging to and intervening in their environment; this, says Jans, is a less adult-centric definition of citizenship: child-sized citizenship.

## CONCEPTUAL FRAMEWORKS

This understanding of citizenship contributes to what has emerged as a new paradigm in sociological studies of childhood (James and Prout, 1990). This conceptual framework advocates for a recognition and inclusion of children's opinions, worldviews, and experiences into all relevant processes–from participatory research to community building. Key viewpoints of this conceptualization include an understanding that "children's social relationships and cultures are worthy of study in their own right, independent of the perspective and concerns of adults," that "children are active in the construction and determination of their own social lives, the lives of those around them and of the societies in which they live," and that ethnography is an effective methodology for the study of childhood as it allows to incorporate their own voice in the production of sociological data (James and Prout, p. 8).

Researchers like William Corsaro apply this perspective by looking at the world through children's eyes: "Socialization is not only a matter of adaptation and internalization but also a process of appropriation, reinvention, and reproduction. Central to this view of socialization is the appreciation of the importance of collective, communal activity–how children negotiate, share, and create culture with adults and each other" (Corsaro, 1997, p. 18). The emphasis is on the mutual relationships and influences among children and between children and adults: children also are active participants in the creation of community and civil society. This is reflected in common behaviors children engage in to evade and at the same time affirm adult-imposed rules, for example.

In his ethnographic research in Italian and United States preschools, Corsaro often found that children were not allowed to bring personal toys to school. The children, however, brought small objects that could be attractive to other children because they were different than those available at the school, and resorted to different strategies to hide them in their pockets and show them to their playmates without catching the teacher's attention. The teachers, aware of the transgression, tended to overlook it since the children's adjustment to the rule avoided the need to constantly enforce it. "Children share and play with smuggled personal objects surreptitiously to avoid detection by the teachers. If the children always played with personal objects in this fashion, there would be no conflict and hence no need for the rule. That is not the case, however, the careful sharing takes place only because the adult rule is in effect. . . . (C)hildren's secondary adjustments often contribute to the maintenance of the adult rules" (Corsaro, pp. 42-43).

In recognizing and seeking children's own voices, therefore, scholars and practitioners applying this sociological perspective affirm children's right to participate and to contribute as full-fledged individuals according to their maturity level and interests. Tracing similarities between children's rights movements and those of women and minorities, they question traditional perspectives that view children as marginal rather than integral to community developments with a limited role as passive recipients of knowledge and care, and promote instead studies and programs that incorporate children as community agents–citizens in their own right.

A key development in the shift towards a more inclusive definition of citizenship has been the 1989 United Nations Convention on the Rights of the Child (CRC), particularly Article 12 which protects children's right to participation and consultation in matters that affect them. The CRC has been the foundation of studies and programs that acknowledge children's voice and capacity to be engaged as social actors in their own right (Devine, 2002) and which have given rise to studies and projects in urban planning that involve children in decision-making. See, for example, Roger Hart's seminal book *Children's Participation: The Theory and Practice of Involving Young Citizens in Community Development and Environmental Care* (1997) and David Driskell's *Creating Better Cities with Children and Youth* (2002).

The CRC seeks to protect children applying a holistic perspective: because they are developing, they are especially vulnerable to disease, malnutrition and poverty, and are affected by policies that do not take their special needs into account. Children do begin their life depending on adults to care for them, but protection is not to be confused with restriction of rights and opportunities to participation. As the youth development approach discussed below shows, the opportunities for participation and decision-making are actually key strategies towards healthy emotional and personal growth. In seeking to recognize children's rights to express views and participate in matters that affect them, the CRC has also led to international agreements that reinforce their need for protection from for example, sexual or labor exploitation and armed conflict (Rajani, 2000).

Another body of knowledge that recognizes young people as active social agents is the positive youth development perspective. This model is the foundation of prevention programs and interventions that shift the attention from "young people as problems to solve" (low academic achievement, teen pregnancy, drugs and alcohol) to a perception of youth as individuals with abilities and positive traits who can succeed if provided with adequate resources and opportunities: relationships with caring adults, activities to build marketable skills, safe places, healthy living, and opportunities to help others (as highlighted in the work developed by America's Promise and the Search Institute). This perspective acknowledges young people's need for adults' support to develop as healthy and responsible persons, while also recognizing their present talents and positive contributions. Humanistic or affective education theories such as those proposed by Daniel Goleman (1995) (emotional intelligence) and Howard Gardner (1983) (multiple intelligences) also encourage more holistic perspectives of the child (or the learner in general), focusing on individual needs and learning styles, rather than on learning problems. Attention to context and experience (rather than solely on logical analysis and information acquisition) is also supported by data emerging from neuroscience research that show the effects of rich interactions with the environment and meaningful personal relationships on brain development such that positive environmental stimulation affects cognitive development. Theories of moral development also show that altruistic attitudes do not occur naturally, but are the product of relevant experiences and relationships with positive role models that display prosocial behavior while also providing opportunities to exercise moral judgment and caring behaviors (Lerner, 2002). Altruism, responsibility, caring and concern for the public good are commonly associated with "the traits of a good citizen."

Richard Lerner (2004) takes this approach further by proposing that development is indeed a matter of relationships and interactions between the young person and his or her social world. "Thriving youth" as defined by Lerner are those who live in a society that offers opportunities to pursue goals and to contribute to their own well-being and the well-being of their communities: "socialization for democracy." Again, the notion of citizenship is viewed through the lens of community-building activities and relationships-participation and appropriation of public life–regardless of age.

In terms of the implications of these conceptual developments for the notion of child-citizens, it is possible to argue that children do many of the same things that adults do when giving meaning to and building communities–a particular dimension of citizenship: They contribute to the economy as students by acquiring the knowledge and skills needed to sustain a society from generation to generation (Qvortrup, 1987), as household members by contributing to the family's sustenance and reproduction by taking care of younger siblings to doing laundry and preparing meals, as volunteers and as young workers. In the political sphere of the school they elect their class or youth group president, debate grades, negotiate assignments, and compromise on length of recess time. In their neighborhoods they use playgrounds or not depending on whether these spaces meet children's standards of safety and enjoyment (often leading adult neighborhood residents to take action if the sites need repairs); they walk through safe tree-lined neighborhoods or on dangerous streets with heavy traffic and no pedestrian walkways. All these activities are part of civil society, making and reproducing a community by using it, establishing connections, transforming it and giving it meaning.

## FELLOW CITIZENS

What do communities look like when the concept of "child-sized citizenship" is applied? The following two examples serve to illustrate this perspective.

The city of Porsgrunn, Norway, incorporates the notion of child citizens as a community principle and a public idea (Pittman, 2002). Children in Porsgrunn are considered *fellow citizens*, a principle included into the city's strategic plan for children and youth. The plan promotes the recognition that "The 5th grade child is an expert at being in 5th grade. This means an attitude towards children as competent individuals and subjects of their own life." In other words, only a 10-year-old has the experience and ability to look at the world through 10-year-old eyes, and therefore they are best suited to offer opinions regarding community issues affecting them. This is directly related to children's rights to participation in matters relevant to their experience and what leads city officials to consult with children when specific issues need to be resolved. The Porsgrunn model represents an effective example of youth-adult partnerships and shared decision-making in community governance.

One such case was the traffic light that officials had prepared to set up at a certain intersection, considering that it was where it was needed the most. The neighborhood children serving on the City Council opposed the measure, indicating that the traffic light was not needed at that intersection but at a different location which children used more frequently and that posed greater risks, and that a speed bump was enough. The solution recommended by the children was implemented, at a lower cost than the original plan and with the desired results (Lillestol, 2004).

Claire Gallagher (2004), a researcher at Georgian Court University in Lakewood, NJ, presents another example of young children participating in the process of community building. Through the "Our Town" project, twenty 8- and 9-year-old urban children designed and built a neighborhood park that satisfied the needs they were concerned about: the design had to facilitate intergenerational interaction, provide safety and be visually pleasing. The initial phase of the project involved the design of a model that took into consideration zoning, infrastructure and other issues, as well as the laws the children wanted enforced– " 'no drugs, no guns, no adults unless . . . ' It was abundantly evident that the children were claiming control of their environment" (p. 253). Once the model was completed, the community was invited to an open house to view the proposed project.

In the second phase, the children mapped their neighborhood and its needs, chose the site for the park, and worked on the actual design proposal. The community was invited to attend bi-weekly meetings to learn about the proposed design and provide input. "As a result of these gatherings," indicates Gallagher, "students became familiar with the preferences and opinions of the other members of the community, but they retained their design objectivity; the adult assumption that the children would design exclusively for themselves was proven unwarranted" (p. 256). During the building phase, the community came together to clear the space, and to build and plant the park. Since it was built, the children monitor and manage the public use of the space, which has served as a place for small concerts and other community events.

Gallagher points out that a possible reason for the positive inter-generational interactions brought about by Our Town, may be found in Hugh Matthews' argument that "policy changes and initiatives designed to foster the inclusion of children in the community design process would result in changes that would benefit both groups" (Gallagher, p. 258). Through the different stages of this project, children displayed a deep understanding of neighborhood issues which were reflected in a park design that met the different generations' needs. The active engagement of children in community design processes, therefore, may be a contributing factor to positive relationships and mutual understanding among the groups involved. Adults' commitment to and confidence in children's capacity to make sound decisions for the community as a whole, emerge as key factors for the possible replication of this case; the Barra Mansa model (described in a later section) presents a similar framework in a different country with comparable results: children given the power to manage a portion of the city budget apply it to projects that serve the whole community's needs.

Both the Porsgrunn and the New Jersey cases are examples of what Jans Marc calls "child-sized citizenship": a status that takes into account the specific ways in which young children participate in and build their communities. These cases also provide specific examples of what Lerner describes as the positive youth development strategies that help youth to flourish and societies to become more democratic through the civic engagement opportunities they provide for young people.

## Different Paths to Child Citizenship

The inter-connected fields of youth service, service-learning and youth in decision-making provide other examples of "children-sized citizenship" through their participation in the life and well-being of their communities, regardless of age. School and community-based initiatives that engage young people in the less conventional roles of active social agents where they are encouraged to assess community needs, as well as design and implement solutions and participate in substantive decisions, are increasingly placing youth in citizen roles no different–although not recognized–than those of adults.

The following program examples, therefore, show the different paths children are adopting to contribute to their communities' well-being and social change.

*Youth-Led Service:* We know that young people are volunteering more than any other generation in the history of the United States, with the 1990s showing the highest volunteering rates among high school students than in the previous five decades (Toppe and Golombek, 2002). Different factors may be contributing to this trend, including the growing number of school districts requiring the completion of service hours for graduation, policies and legislation encouraging youth service, a cooperative attitude as a characteristic of the millennial generation (Howe and Strauss, 2000), and a general inclination to help others and to rebuild communities after the events of September 11, 2001.

Around the world, this trend towards increased participation in service activities is also clear. Countries participating in Global Youth Service Day, an annual global campaign to highlight the contributions of youth to their communities, have grown from 27 when it was launched in 2000 to over 100 participating countries in 2005.

- *AstroTots*: Rebecca Robison (age 13, from Layton, UT) created a space camp for girls ages 4 to 10, based on a teacher-led program for older youth. "AstroTots; Space Camp for Little Dippers," a 3 hour "camp" organized on special youth service days such as National Youth Service Day (April 16-18, 2004), provides fun activities for little girls to learn about and become interested in space science. "The first improvement I feel I made in my community," says Becca, "is getting other kids excited about community service and now starting projects of their own. Also, girls have learned more about science and that science is an option in their futures." Becca, with the help of youth and adult volunteers trained in specific topics, runs similar camps on other science subjects such as "Love Bugs: Insects, Bugs, and Crawly Friends" and "Mad Female Scientists" (*www.astrotots.org*).
- *Kidz Voice-LA*: Concerned with the number of youth shot in Los Angeles, CA, then 11-year-old twin brothers Theo and Niko Milonopoulos co-founded in 1998 Kidz Voice-LA, a non-profit organization to provide youth with a voice in public policy and to lobby for gun control legislation in the city. Through petitions, attendance at anti-gun violence marches, public speeches, and testimonies, Kidz Voice-LA has helped change the city's gun policy. The youth-led organization coordinated a gun meltdown rally with

the Police Department and successfully lobbied the Los Angeles City Council to pass a partial ban on ammunition sales.

*Service-Learning:* Service-learning is an educational approach that combines academic subject learning with community service. Through this model, children make connections between curricular topics and their application in community settings. The service addresses a true community need identified by the youth themselves, and also meets academic standards. A reflection component embedded in the process encourages youth to analyze their service experience and understand larger community issues. Service-learning critics question the effectiveness of the approach when it is mandated. However, while more research is required, studies conducted to date indicate that service-learning methodologies do indeed lead to positive outcomes. "Service-learning–partly through its effects on students' sense of community and positive school climate–may especially help to increase the engagement and motivation of disadvantaged students. Brandeis University researchers found that service-learning's academic and civic impact was greater for lower income, minority, and more at-risk youth" (Scales and Roehlkepartain, 2005, p. 15). Other studies show that overall positive effects of service-learning can be found in students' cognitive skills, their sense of connection to society and community, their personal and interpersonal development, and career exploration skills (Billig, 2004, p. 14). Other studies have also shown that an emotional connection to the topic studied (as achieved through meaningful experiential learning), leads to increased learning, which would lend support to service-learning models.

- *Voter Registration Drive:* As part of a social studies unit on the 1996 presidential election, eighth grade students at Great Falls Middle Schools in Montague, MA conducted a voter registration drive on the village green and other public places. They set up booths with signs that read "Vote for me Today; I'll Vote for you Tomorrow," passed out flags, information about the candidates and about key election issues, and voter registration forms and instructions. The teacher, Lisa Greco, stressed the value of this particular project in a community that was not politically active. In addition, the survey the children conducted allowed the students to see where their community stood on different issues while enabling the community to see the children in a citizenship role (Roberts, 2002).

- *"Ecoleños":* Ruca Antu School is a school for students with special needs, located in Junin de los Andes, a very poor town in southern Argentina. In 2001, challenged by the reality of very cold winters and scarce heating resources, students researched different forms of alternative energy. Testing different options and comparing caloric yield, they discovered that they could produce an efficient heating source by compacting balls of wet paper and other organic materials. The result was "Ecoleños" or ecological logs. Today, after continuing to learn about the product and the heating process, the mixture has been improved to include paper, potato peals, dried leaves and other items. Furthermore, the children have trained their own families, neighbors, and students in regular schools in the use of the logs as an efficient and environmentally friendly heating alternative as they also educate others on paper recycling strategies (*http://www.comunidar.org.ar/premioashoka 2.htm*).

*Youth in Philanthropy:* Through youth philanthropy programs young people are incorporated into grant-making boards, often affiliated with community foundations and overseeing community development projects. Youth philanthropy trains young people to identify community problems and design the most appropriate solutions in a systematic way (Cretsinger, n.d.). Experience in youth philanthropy programs shows that young philanthropists tend to offer creative ways to solve problems, go beyond the grant-making to offer their time, and support efforts that address community-wide issues and not just those focused on youth (an experience similar to the example provided by Gallagher in "Our Town" project).

- *Penny Harvest Campaign:* Through its Penny Harvest Program, Common Cents New York engages students ages 4 to 18 in allocating funds to community projects. Starting with a penny recycling program, every New York City school that collects enough pennies to fill 25 sacks is eligible for a Student Roundtable grant of $1,000. Common Cents trains teachers in qualifying schools to run a 12-16 week philanthropy Roundtable for student leaders, grades K-12. Teams of students cooperatively assess their communities' needs, pay site visits to neighborhood organizations, review proposals and award grants. Students have provided over $500,000 in grants to beautify communities, save animals, pay for medical supplies, support AIDS education campaigns and other global relief projects. The program's greatest accomplishment is that it teaches students that their voices matter and their actions can effect real change.

- *High School Philanthropists:* The Michigan Women's Foundation Young Women for Change program and the Winnipeg Foundation's Youth in Philanthropy program represent two examples of collaboration between foundations and local high schools. Through the Young Women for Change program, 14- to 18-year-old girls from diverse geographic, socio-economic and ethnic backgrounds are selected by their peers to serve two-year terms on the foundation's grantmaking committee. The young women implement the entire grantmaking process, from writing the Request for Proposals to conducting site visits and selecting final recipients. Each committee grants up to $20,000 annually to nonprofit groups serving the needs of young women and girls in their geographic area. The program's focus on gender issues addresses the need for increased funding for women and girls as well as the young philanthropists' of gender-based socio-economic problems (*www.miwf.org*).

- *Youth in Philanthropy*, an initiative of The Winnipeg Foundation in Canada, allocates funds for high-school based Youth Advisory Committees to distribute to causes of their choice. Students discuss their committees' values and goals, research possible recipients and decide how to allocate funds. Projects funded by the youth in 2003 included software and educational videos for residents with disabilities, equipment for several health clinics and workshops and training on sexual abuse prevention, youth employment and inter-cultural communication.

*Youth in Decision-Making:* The notion of young people's involvement in decision-making addresses their role in determining the outcomes of any project or initiative. While still infrequent overall, a growing number of youth organizations and agencies are incorporating young people into youth advisory councils and boards of directors, with positive results. Zeldin, McDaniel, Topitzes and Calvert (2000) conducted a study of fifteen organizations that incorporate 12 to 21 year olds either on their board of directors or in program decision-making. Results from this study indicate overall positive outcomes including an improved perception of youth by adults, greater commitment of adults to the organization, a stronger focus on the organizational mission, and a greater value placed on diversity and representation.

Examples of activities conducted by youth in a decision-making role include Youth Service America's governing board which incorporates four youth members with full voting privileges. An alternative to the formal juvenile justice system, Youth Courts around the country involve 8 to 18 year olds in judging and sentencing peers for first-time crimes, traffic or school rule violations. An Urban Institute study of teen courts found peer pressure to be a positive strategy to help young offenders understand the impact of their behaviors as well indications of lower rates of recidivism in youth courts. The Youth Council of the City of Hampton, Virginia, consists of 24 high school-age youth who represent young people's views on city issues and acts in an advisory capacity to the City Council. Their activities include rewriting the city's bicycle ordinance and assisting in the development of a city-wide bikeway system; they also awarded $100,000 to youth-led projects and succeeded in including a teen center in city plans.

A number of factors contribute to the degree of effectiveness of these initiatives. A positive perception of youth rather than as problems is critical, since without an appreciation of youths' talents and contributions, power-sharing would not be possible. At the same time the stronger the internalization of this attitude at the highest leadership level, the more successful the inclusion of youth will be. Significant training is also recommended both for adults and youth to make these youth-adult interactions successful as in many cases, the inclusion of youth as partners requires a cultural shift from traditional ways of operating.

City planning is also an area where there are attempts to include children as decision-makers. This is an effective and direct strategy to engage children in the design and planning of the environment in which they live, study, work and play. As stated by the Porsgrunn council described above, "ten year olds are experts at being ten years old" and therefore know better than anyone else what their needs are and how to address them from an urban planning perspective.

- *Democracy in School:* The Fairhaven School in Upper Marlboro, Maryland is a private school which promotes democratic principles among its student body, administration, parents and faculty. The governing body of the school is the Assembly, composed of parents, students, staff and community members. It sets major policies, amends by-laws, sets annual tuition, makes budget allocations and awards diplomas. Day-to-day decisions are made by the School Meeting which gathers weekly to manage all the school affairs. Every student from 5 to 18 and all regular staff are full members of the Meeting with an equal vote in all decisions. Meetings are run by an elected Chair according to Robert's Rules of Order and recorded by a secretary. The school meeting makes rules about the conduct of its members, elects staff annually, and runs operations by committees such as Admissions, Bookkeeping, Grounds Maintenance, and Public Relations. Anyone is eligible to serve on these committees. Positions which require greater experience or specific knowledge such as Bookkeeping Clerk are usually held by staff members. The Judicial Committee is given the responsibility for enforcing school rules and it is the only committee on which every member of the School Meeting must serve. A tendency is for older students to help and look out for younger ones, establishing a sense of camaraderie across age groups. "The school's democracy achieves that subtle balance between individual rights and community responsibility and creates the environment of fairness, tolerance and respect which each of us seeks and deserves."

- *Participatory Budgeting:* The Children's Participatory Budget Council in Barra Mansa, Brazil, was established in 1998 to foster citizenship among children and youth between 9 and 15 years old. The children elect 18 boys and 18 girls from among their peers to a children's council, which manages a portion of the municipal budget (about US$ 125,000) to be used according to the council's priorities. Every year since its inception, the council has allotted funds to projects such as school repairs and equipment, better security and improved playgrounds in low-income areas, repairs of sewers and drains, and tree planting. Specific projects the child councilors are especially proud of are a new all-weather sports surface at the municipal school, the lighting of the Pombal Tunnel in one of the central neighborhoods where children play in the evenings and the renovation of a health clinic. The young councilors are gaining the skills to take on active roles in meetings of the city councilors and residents' associations. As one child phrased it "We can't imagine that only adults have a say in the running of our city." The opportunity to work with public budgets and to represent their peers' interests is Barra Mansa's strategy to affirming young people's "rightful status as full citizens" (Guerra, 2002).

These cases represent only a few examples of the multiple ways in which children exercise citizenship through community participation.

Both Astrotots and Kidz Voice-LA are youth-led service initiatives, that utilize different approaches and scale: Astrotots targets a specific constituency at the local level (an identified need for greater involvement of girls in science) while Kidz Voice-LA seeks to change public policy at the city level regarding gun control. The Children's Participatory Budget Council of Barra Mansa also enables children to affect local government policy, but in this case through actual budget management. The Fairhaven School experience replicates this model at the school level, engaging students, teachers and administrators as equal partners in school management. The examples of youth philanthropy educate and engage young children and high school students to assess community needs and allocate funds to carefully selected projects; experiences sharpen their analytical and decision-making skills and as research shows are the foundation for lifelong participation in philanthropic activities. Finally, the case of the ecological logs project in Argentina and the voter registration drive in Massachusetts allowed children to successfully play non-traditional roles as teachers and activists.

The cases described above have different approaches and scales; they range from individual efforts to government initiatives, and from classroom projects to radical experiments in school democracy. What is common about them, however, is the positioning of children in roles usually considered as adult domains: teachers, philanthropists, budget managers, advocates.

## IMPLICATIONS AND BARRIERS TO CHILDREN'S PARTICIPATION

Participation in these different forms of service activities offers children opportunities to learn new skills. From public speaking to partnership building, from negotiating to fundraising, and from deciding on conflicting community priorities to managing their time, are all skills that can be acquired through participation in activities such as those described. However, there is also a risk in viewing these activities as only *preparation for the future*, and not recognizing children as citizens in the here and now. "To assert that children learn about citizenship through participation is tantamount to the 'human becomings' argument, so that children's citizenship, exercised through democratic processes is in danger of only being valuable because of the citizens they will become. By not being given its proper place as an essential stage in human society, childhood is thus diminished" (Ennew, 2000).

Having noted the potential for children's participation, it is clear that barriers to their engagement still exist. Among those barriers are organizational cultures or adult attitudes that may prevent thinking about children in new roles; in other words, a lack of adult awareness that the way we relate to children is socially constructed, defined by history and geography, and can change. Barriers to children's involvement can also take the form of programs that do not take into account their school schedules, homework commitments, and special needs for transportation, for example. The issue of possible liabilities and legal concerns is also considered an obstacle to involving children in less traditional roles.

There are, however, many resources and opportunities to lift barriers such as these. Organizations and schools committed to engaging children in more participatory programs, for example, can prepare all stakeholders through trainings and open discussions about stereotypes, exercises in "shared power" and listening to children's ideas, decision-making processes that incorporate their perspectives, and logistical arrangements that meet children's needs and schedules. Organizations such as Youth on Board, Innovation Center and 4H offer trainings, technical assistance, and resources on these issues.

Liability concerns need to be addressed by consulting child labor laws, insurance carriers, and ensuring that children are engaged in safe activities; adults and children need to be aware of risk management procedures, although neither children nor adults would be placed in risk situations in the first place. But the possibility of a liability concern cannot be raised as a barrier to children's participation without also considering established practices that facilitate their involvement (Toppe and Golombek, 2002).

From a family perspective, opportunities for parents and children to engage in civic activities together also contribute to lifting the barriers presented by traditional parent-child roles and encourages family members to work as a team and see each other in a new light (Toppe and Golombek, 2002). Resources and "how to" guides such as Jenny Friedman's The Busy Family Guide to Volunteering (2003) present options to engage children along with their families in projects that range from direct service to people in need, to social action, political engagement, and environmental activism, and in every case advocating that there are age-appropriate activities available for all children once the commitment to their engagement has been made. See also Teaching Your Kids to Care by Deborah Spaide (1995), who argues that "Adults have been involving kids in fund-raising drives for decades. What is new is empowering kids to be the leaders in social change" (p. 11).

Finally, educational systems and teachers socialized to engage children in roles beyond that of passive students–through meaningful service-learning methodologies, for example–also open up new avenues and lift traditional obstacles to children's civic participation.

## CONCLUSION

"City's gun policy changed." "Science camp for little girls." "Budget approved for community projects." These could easily be headlines in local newspapers and readers would not hesitate in associating these projects with civic endeavors led, by adult citizens. However, as the examples provided in this article show, these and thousands of other projects are being created, led, and organized by young children every day in this country and around the world.

A recognition of these activities as important contributions to civic life by the youngest residents implies a shift in our understanding of what is true democracy: a system in which each member is recognized for the skills they have at a specific maturational stage and that, as Richard Lerner argues, offers quality opportunities to contribute those skills and opinions to the common good.

Deep cultural changes are required for a society to view and incorporate young children as active citizens. There needs to be a recognition that children and their cultures are subjects of study and programming in their own right, independent of adult perspectives and interests. In other words, it must be accepted that young children are not just passive recipients of adult social structures but actively construct their own lives and the lives of those around them (James and Prout, 1990). Acceptance of this perspective leads to the recognition that children have their own experiences and unique view of the world, and that communities become healthier when children's rights to participation are protected and encouraged. This attitude also implies attention to what children *can* do at different maturational states, rather than on what they cannot do (either because of biological immaturity or socially-constructed restrictions). In this sense, truly democratic and representative societies would be those where citizenship is defined by the connection and interdependencies among all members, even the youngest ones, each making their own contributions to healthier and more sustainable communities.

# REFERENCES

America's Promise, The Alliance for Youth. (n.d.). *The five promises*. Retrieved May 25, 2005, from http://www.americaspromise.org/whyhere/5promises.cfm

Billig, S. (2004). Heads, hearts, and hands: The research on K-12 service-learning. In *Growing to Greatness 2004* (pp.12-25). St. Paul: National Youth Leadership Council.

Corsaro, W. (1997). *The sociology of childhood*. Thousand Oaks, CA: Pine Forge Press.

Cretsinger, M. (n.d.). Youth philanthropy: A framework of best practice. Retrieved May 25, 2005, from Kellogg Foundation website: www.wkkf.org/Pubs/PhilVol/Pub557.pdf

Devine, D. (2002). Children's citizenship and the structuring of adult-child relations in the primary school. *Childhood: A Global Journal of Child Research, 9*, 303-320.

Driskell, D. (2002). *Creating better cities with children and youth: A manual for participation*. London: UNESCO Publishing.

Ennew, J. (2000). *How can we define citizenship in childhood?* Revised and extended version of a presentation at the Seminar on the Political Participation of Children, Harvard University Center for Population and Development Studies, May 1999.

Friedman, J. (2003). *The busy family's guide to volunteering*. Beltsville, MD: Robins Lane Press.

Gallagher, C. (2004). "Our Town": Children as advocates for change in the city. *Childhood, A Global Journal of Child Research, 11*, 251-262.

Gardner, H. (1983). *Frames of mind: The theory of multiple intelligences*. New York: BasicBooks.

Goleman, D. (1995). *Emotional intelligence: Why it can matter more than IQ*. New York: Bantam Books.

Guerra, E. (2002). Citizenship knows no age: Children's participation in the governance and municipal budget of Barra Mansa, Brazil. *Environment and Urbanization, 14*, 71-84.

Hart, R. (1997). *Children's participation: The theory and practice of involving young citizens in community development and environmental care*. London: Earthscan.

Howe, N., & Strauss, W. (2000). *Millennials rising: The next great generation*. New York: Vintage Books.

James, A., & Prout, A. (Eds.). (1990). *Constructing and reconstructing childhood: Contemporary issues in the sociological study of childhood*. New York: The Falmer Press.

Jans, M. (2004). Children as citizens: Towards a contemporary notion of child participation. *Childhood: A Global Journal of Child Research, 11*, 27-44.

Lerner, R. (2002). *Adolescence: Development, diversity, context, and application*. New Jersey: Pearson Education.

Lerner, R. (2004). *Liberty: Thriving and civic engagement among America's youth*. Thousand Oaks: Sage Publications.

Lillestol, K. (2004). *Service-learning in Europe*. Presentation at the National Service Learning Conference, Orlando, Fl., March 2004. (More information on the Posgrunn model can be found at *http://www.lillestol.no/english/index.php*)

Patrick, J. (n.d.). *The concept of citizenship in education for democracy.* Retrieved May 25, 2005, from ERIC Digest: http://www.ericdigests.org/2000-1/democracy.html

Pittman, K. (2002). Balancing the equation: Communities supporting youth, youth supporting communities. *CYD Anthology,* 19-24.

Qvortrup, J. (1987). The sociology of childhood: Introduction. *International Journal of Sociology, 17,* 3-37

Rajani, R. (2000, Summer). Introduction: How do we think about children. *Cultural Survival Quarterly,* 41-43.

Roberts, P. (2002). *Kids taking action: Community service learning projects K-8.* Greenfield: Northeast Foundation for Children.

Scales, P. & Roehlkepartain, E. (2005). Can service-learning help reduce the achievement gap? New research points toward the potential of service-learning for low-income students. *Growing to Greatness 2005* (pp.10-22). St. Paul: National Youth Leadership Council.

Search Institute. (n.d.). Introduction to assets. Retrieved May 25, 2005, from http://www.search-institute.org/assets/

Spaide, D. (1995). *Teaching your kids to care: How to discover and develop the spirit of charity in your children.* New York: Carol Publishing Group.

Toppe, C., & Golombek, S. (2002). *Engaging youth in lifelong service: Findings and recommendations for encouraging a tradition of voluntary action among America's youth.* Washington, DC: Independent Sector.

Zeldin, S., McDaniel A., Topitzes, D., & Calvert, A. (2000). Youth in decision-making: A study on the impacts of youth on adults and organizations. Chevy Chase: The Innovation Center for Community and Youth Development.

# Toward a Critical Social Theory
# of Youth Empowerment

Louise B. Jennings, PhD
Deborah M. Parra-Medina, MPH, PhD
DeAnne K. Hilfinger Messias, PhD, RN
Kerry McLoughlin, MA

**SUMMARY.** This article contributes to the development of a critical social theory of youth empowerment which emphasizes collective efforts to create sociopolitical change. It draws upon analysis of four youth empowerment models, and upon findings from a participatory research

---

Louise B. Jennings is Associate Professor, Department of Educational Psychology, University of South Carolina, Columbia, SC 29208 (E-mail: ljenning@gwm.sc.edu). Deborah M. Parra-Medina is Associate Professor, Department of Health Promotion, Education, and Behavior, Arnold School of Public Health, and Women's Studies Department, University of South Carolina, Columbia, SC 29208 (E-mail: dpmedina@ sc.edu). DeAnne K. Hilfinger Messias is Associate Professor, College of Nursing and Women's Studies Program, University of South Carolina, 201 Flinn Hall, Columbia, SC 29208. Kerry McLoughlin is Qualitative Research Analyst, Family Health International, Durham, NC 27713 (E-mail: kmcloughlin@fhi.org).

The authors acknowledge the contributions of Elizabeth Fore, Sherer Royce, and Terry Williams.

This manuscript was developed through a grant from the American Legacy Foundation with collaboration from the CDC Foundation, and scientific and technical assistance from the Centers for Disease Control and Prevention. The Grantee's Informational Materials do not necessarily represent the views of the American Legacy Foundation or the CDC Foundation, their respective Staff or their respective Board of Directors.

[Haworth co-indexing entry note]: "Toward a Critical Social Theory of Youth Empowerment." Jennings, Louise B. et al. Co-published simultaneously in *Journal of Community Practice* (The Haworth Press, Inc.) Vol. 14, No. 1/2, 2006, pp. 31-55; and: *Youth Participation and Community Change* (ed: Barry N. Checkoway, and Lorraine M. Gutiérrez) The Haworth Press, Inc., 2006, pp. 31-55. Single or multiple copies of this article are available for a fee from The Haworth Document Delivery Service [1-800-HAWORTH, 9:00 a.m. - 5:00 p.m. (EST). E-mail address: docdelivery@haworthpress.com].

study which identified key dimensions of critical youth empowerment: (1) a welcoming, safe environment, (2) meaningful participation and engagement, (3) equitable power-sharing between youth and adults, (4) engagement in critical reflection on interpersonal and sociopolitical processes, (5) participation in sociopolitical processes to affect change, and (6) integrated individual- and community-level empowerment. It concludes with discussion of the measurement of outcomes, and the challenges and opportunities for empowerment in youth organization.

**KEYWORDS.** Youth, youth empowerment, model development, participatory research, critical social theory

## INTRODUCTION

Efforts to support youths' healthy development and integration into the community have experienced several shifts in focus over the past few decades (Small, 2004). Historically, a primary function of youth programs was rehabilitation or containment (e.g., keeping youth off the streets). An initial shift from these risk-based preventive approaches was in the direction of fostering healthy youth development and capacity building through active community participation (Kim, 1998; Small, 2004). More recently, positive youth development approaches have been expanded to incorporate a focus on youth empowerment.

Empowerment is a multi-level construct consisting of practical approaches and applications, social action processes, and individual and collective outcomes. In the broadest sense, empowerment refers to individuals, families, organizations, and communities gaining control and mastery, within the social, economic, and political contexts of their lives, in order to improve equity and quality of life (Rappaport, 1984; Rappaport, 1987; Zimmerman, 2000). The concept of empowerment has been addressed at both theoretical and practice levels in specific reference to youth.

The aim of this paper is to contribute toward the development of a critical social theory of youth empowerment. We begin with a theoretical overview of empowerment and an examination of four conceptual models of youth empowerment identified through an extensive review of the literature, from multiple disciplinary perspectives. While recognizing that additional research examines dimensions of youth empowerment and informs our analysis of these models (e.g., Heath, 1991; Heath, 1994), we focused our search and examination specifically on conceptual models of youth empowerment.

Drawing on our analysis of these existing models and our participatory research, we identify and discuss six essential dimensions of Critical Youth Empowerment (CYE). We propose CYE as a conceptual framework based on the integration of youth empowerment processes and outcomes at the individual and collective levels. These occur within welcoming, youth-centered environments, through meaningful engagement and knowledge, skill, and leadership development, critical reflection on societal forces and power relations, and active community participation, leading to change in sociopolitical processes, structures, norms, or images. The final sections present our discussion of the challenges and opportunities for incorporating the dimensions of CYE within youth organizations, issues of measurement, and potential benefits of CYE for youth and communities.

## MODELS OF YOUTH EMPOWERMENT

Empowerment is a social action process that can occur at multiple levels, e.g., individual, family, organization, and community. Theorists and researchers across multiple disciplines have examined and analyzed empowerment and linked it to individual and collective health, well-being, and environments (Freire, 1970; Jones, 1993; Pinderhughes, 1995; Rappaport, 1987; Wallerstein, 1992; Zimmerman, 1988). Rocha (1997) proposed empowerment as a continuum or ladder, with Atomistic Individual Empowerment (focus on changing the individual) and Political Empowerment (focus on changing the community) as the two endpoints. Such a continuum focuses on only one dimension of empowerment–the level or subject (individual vs. collective). At the individual level, psychological empowerment focuses on individual-level capacity-building, integrating perceptions of personal control, a proactive approach to life, and a critical understanding of the sociopolitical environment (Zimmerman, 1995; Zimmerman, 2000). Collective empowerment occurs within families, organizations, and communities, involving processes and structures that enhance members' skills, provide them with mutual support necessary to effect change, improve their collective well-being, and strengthen intra-

and inter-organizational networks and linkages to improve or maintain the quality of community life.

Conceptualizing youth empowerment as a bipolar continuum does not reflect other key dimensions of this complex social action process, such as the philosophy and values underlying youth programs and initiatives, the dynamics of youth-adult relationships within these initiatives, and individual and collective processes of critical reflection and reflective action to address social injustice and inequities. Rissel (1994) emphasized the integrated and sociopolitical dimensions of empowerment, noting that "community empowerment includes a raised level of psychological empowerment among its members, a political action component in which members have actively participated, and the achievement of some redistribution of resources or decision making favorable to the community or group in question" (p. 41). In the following sections we examine four models, both theoretical and practice-based, that have been developed to explain and guide youth empowerment efforts within communities.

### Adolescent Empowerment Cycle

The Adolescent Empowerment Cycle (AEC) is a model developed by Chinman and Linney (1998). The AEC is based on psychological theories of adolescent development and describes processes aimed at preventing a sense of rolelessness and enhance self-esteem. Chinman and Linney linked AEC to the developmental process of social bonding, leading youth to bond to positive institutions through action, skill development, and reinforcement. Positive social bonding can prevent youth engagement in negative social activities. Given its theoretical basis, the AEC centers on three dimensions: *adolescent participation in meaningful activities*, such as community service, that provide *opportunities for skill development* and *positive reinforcement and recognition from adults* throughout the process. The authors argued that for adolescents experiencing a period of identity crisis and formation, participation in meaningful activity may contribute to role stability, offsetting a general lack of purpose or direction many adolescents experience.

Chinman and Linney (1998) offered the example of older high school students mentoring incoming freshmen regarding their transition to high school as an illustration of how the processes of the AEC might be realized. They noted that participation in peer mentoring activities could provide adolescents with meaningful roles and organizational and communication skills that will be useful in later life. Positive recognition by adults of the youth mentoring roles and activities would have beneficial implications for youths' maturing self-esteem and self-efficacy. However, the authors did not provide details about youths' roles and responsibilities nor did they describe how adults engage in this process with positive reinforcement, a critical feature of the AEC model.

## Youth Development and Empowerment Program Model

The aim of the Youth Development and Empowerment (YD&E) is to guide youth empowerment initiatives within the context of substance abuse prevention programs (Kim, 1998). Similar to the AEC model, the YD&E goes beyond the prevention of risky behaviors and is based on meaningful participation of youth in community service projects. A key to the YD&E process is the enhancement of positive social bonding and preparation for participation and involvement in the socioeconomic and public affairs of the community. The model is grounded in social control theory, social learning theory, and expectations-states theory.

In their presentation and discussion of the YD&E model, Kim and colleagues (1998) described the features of youth empowerment processes and specified core structural components that support these processes. The model explicitly incorporates dimensions of both individual empowerment and community engagement, or community partnership. The central tenet of YD&E is the recognition that youth are assets and resources that should be called upon to participate in community and social affairs. However, the YD&E process requires strong social support from caring and supportive adults who place high expectations on youth participants and reinforce achievement. The authors envisioned participation in youth-determined community service projects as meaningful opportunities for youth to learn life skills that have vocational implications, take responsibility, and demonstrate their abilities and success. The accomplishments also need to be recognized and celebrated by significant others in the community.

Within the YD&E model, the role of the adult leader is to serve as a guide and facilitator, allowing the youth leader to take on leadership responsibility for the ensuing activities. As projects are completed, participants evaluate their efforts, determine future directions, recognize everyone's contributions, and celebrate their success. Desired youth outcomes include the development of positive relationships with both peers and adults, participation in social/public affairs, and demonstration of success in solving real community problems and issues (Kim et al., 1998).

As an example of a context for the realization of the YD&E process, Kim and colleagues (1998) described youth participation in a community-based task force made up of representatives from social agencies and organizations. The task force would provide leadership, expertise and community resources to youth teams engaged in community service projects. The teams would be led by youth-adult pairs trained in core skills, such as team-building, communication, problem-solving, and interpersonal social skills. In turn, the youth-adult dyads would train youth team members in the same core skills as they work together to develop team-determined service projects. Ideally, such projects would have career-building potential and address local social concerns (e.g., a drug-free public awareness campaign, an anti-tobacco media promotion). In the process, youth members would practice the core skills while creating, planning, and evaluating their activities with shared responsibilities. When needed, youth teams would draw upon the sponsoring task forces for further training and support. Youth participation in making regular presentations to the task forces would serve to send an ongoing message that youth are important and valued by the community and also reinforce youth achievements.

### The Transactional Partnering Model

A longitudinal qualitative study of a community-based youth empowerment program in Canada resulted in the development of a Transactional Partnering (TP) model (Cargo 2003). An inner-city community health promotion intervention aimed at youth engagement with local quality of life (QOL) issues was the context of this research project. The study examined the process of adult practitioners supporting youth participants in assessing their own QOL issues, developing action plans, and implementing solutions. In contrast to the AEC and YD&E models, which were based on existing theories of youth development and psychology, the TP model of youth empowerment was developed as part of a qualitative research project. However, there are some similarities and overlap across these models.

In the TP model, youth empowerment is conceptualized as a mutual process of transactional partnering between adults and youth (Cargo et al., 2003). Key to this process is the role of adults in creating an empowering and welcoming environment and facilitating and enabling youth. The findings from the qualitative research described various ways in which adults enabled youth. These included ensuring youth had the skills and knowledge they needed to participate in community change efforts through adult facilitating, teaching, mentoring, and providing feedback. One strategy adult facilitators used was to provide youth participants with a roadmap to guide their assessment of QOL issues, develop action plans, and implement solutions. The researchers noted that over time, "adults incrementally gave up responsibility for voicing, decision making, and action, making it available for youth to take" (p. S70). Adult practitioners apparently needed to determine the amount of support required "without undermining the very autonomy enablement is intended to foster" (p. S70) and incrementally transferred responsibility and decision making power to youth as they gained competence and confidence.

Another central tenet of the TP model is the notion of the inter-relatedness of individual and community-level empowerment outcomes. Youth are expected to experience individual outcomes incrementally through participation and success in community change efforts. These outcomes include increased self- and community-esteem, confidence, and competencies such as voicing one's opinion and leadership. Participants also achieve community-level empowerment and develop participatory competence, or the ability to work successfully with others through cooperation, compromise, and appreciation. Youth control is manifest through youth taking responsibility, voicing their opinions, making decisions, and taking action to achieve their goal. The TP model reflects the premise that exposing youth to opportunities and challenges within a safe and supportive environment, and the resulting engagement and reflection, can result in learning and empowerment (Cargo et al., 2003).

In describing the context of the research from which the TP model developed, the authors did not provide descriptions of specific youth activities, projects, or organizational outcomes. However, they outlined processes that supported youth empowerment, defined as "healthful adaptation of youth to confronting challenges associated with directing a youth-defined agenda" (Cargo et al., p. S73). The researchers observed a variety of youth outcomes, including positive self-attributions (self-esteem) and group attributions (collective esteem) in response to achieving success; expressions of increasing confidence over time; evidence of clearer understanding of the workings of local community affairs (raised consciousness); development of voice and advocacy competencies by "talking with greater openness in a group of peers and adults" (p. S75); and increased participatory competence (e.g., cooperating, compromising, appreciating diverse viewpoints, and abandoning stereotypes). The authors argued that TP supported not only youth development (e.g., autonomy, identity, expansion of life chances) but also opportunities to become more socially integrated into the community.

## The Empowerment Education Model

Working with community adult literacy programs in Brazil, Freire (1970) developed and applied his theories of critical social praxis. The premise of his work is that liberating and empowering education is a process that involves listening, dialogue, critical reflection, and reflective action. Freirian concepts of conscientization, liberation, praxis, and empowerment education have been incorporated into various health education initiatives and models. In developing a youth empowerment model for an adolescent health program, Wallerstein, Sanchez-Merki, and Velarde (2005) linked Freirian concepts and practices with protection-motivation behavior change theory. The resulting Empowerment Education (EE) model specifically emphasizes the development of skills and knowledge that support youth efforts toward social action and change and links individual empowerment to community organizing. The authors envisioned the ultimate outcomes of the EE processes as increased self-, collective-, and political-efficacy, resulting in both self-protective individual behaviors as well as other-protective socially responsible behaviors. By fostering the development of empathy and active participation in critical analysis of societal forces within a safe group context, EE can bridge individual behavior change and group efforts for social change.

The EE model guided the development and implementation of a community health prevention program serving predominantly Native American, Hispanic, and low-income Anglo communities in New Mexico (Wallerstein, Sanchez-Merki, & Velarde, 2005). The program offered small groups of youth the opportunities to interview and interact with hospital patients and prison inmates with personal experiences related to drug, tobacco, and alcohol abuse, interpersonal violence, HIV infection, and other high-risk behaviors. The program facilitators were trained university graduate students who followed an extensive curriculum and engaged youth in a Freirian listening-dialogue-action-reflection cycle. The EE process involved story-telling, listening, and sharing of life experiences between the youth and the hospital patients and prison residents. These personal interviews and interactions were followed by participation in group sessions of structured reflection and discussion revolving around the personal, social, medical, and legal consequences of risky behaviors, and the exploration of action strategies to help participants make "healthier choices for themselves and their communities" (p. 220).

Through these dialogue cycles, youth engaged in critical reflection, or conscientization, analyzing the societal context for personal problems and their own role in working on the problems. Protection-motivation variables were integrated throughout the dialogue cycles. For example, as youth listened to the patients' and prison residents' stories, the EE processes facilitated cognitive awareness of precursors to and consequences of alcohol problems, leading youth to conduct a personal coping appraisal. Facilitators also used an inductive questioning guide in order to engage youth in different levels of critical thinking and help participants acquire beliefs in their ability to help themselves and others. Participants engaged in dialogue about their own personal lives, relationships, and communities and were guided to develop an awareness of school and neighborhood resources in order to build socially responsible behaviors. Facilitators led the dialogue sessions but also engaged with youth as "co-learners," offering youth the experience of contributing to adults' learning through their participation.

The aim of youth participation in these interactions, reflections, and dialogues was praxis, "an ongoing interaction between reflection and the actions that people take to promote individual and community change" (Wallerstein, Sanchez-Merki, & Velarde, 2005, p. 221). Toward the end of the program, youth moved from reflection to action by engaging in community action projects. Participants chose to engage in presentations and peer teaching or in community-based organizing, such as production of "community murals, and ethnic-cultural institutes that reflected their community, culture and the voice of local youths" (2005, p. 225). Other examples of the outcomes of the EE processes included the creation of videos for use in educational efforts in neighborhood schools and community centers and a local youth-produced series of television programs on teen life. Several participants also joined with larger community initiatives to develop tobacco policy recommendations.

In summary, our examination of these four models yields a composite view of youth empowerment. As underscored in the AEC and YD&E models, youth empowerment involves a participatory cycle that engages youth in a safe environment and meaningful activities where they can learn skills, confront challenges, demonstrate success, and receive support and positive reinforcement for their efforts, can lead to empowerment on an individual level. The YD&E model also emphasizes the importance of youth serving in leadership roles, although this is limited to those youth paired with adult leaders of the task forces. The TP model captures the attribute of shared power among adults and youth members to a greater degree than the other models. It also offers a process for developing youth-led community-change activities that provide all youth participants with leadership opportunities. Finally, by emphasizing critical reflection and structural level change, the EE model represents specific components of youth empowerment that distinguish it from the other models.

## TOWARD A CRITICAL SOCIAL THEORY OF YOUTH EMPOWERMENT

Critical social theories are interdisciplinary in origin and focus on emancipatory processes that give rise to community actions and the promotion of social justice (Campbell, 1991). To further critical social theory and practice around youth empowerment, we propose that critical youth empowerment (CYE) encompasses those processes and contexts through which youth engage in actions that create change in organizational, institutional, and societal policies, structures, values, norms, and images. CYE builds on, integrates, and expands existing conceptual models of youth development and youth empowerment. The aim of CYE is to support and foster youth contributions to positive community development and sociopolitical change, resulting in youth who are critical citizens, actively participating in the day-to-day building of stronger, more equitable communities (Jennings & Green, 1993).

We bring to this discussion the findings from our participatory research with community youth organizations (Messias, Fore, McLoughlin, & Parra-Medina, 2005; Royce, 2004; Royce, April 2004). The research . was developed within a community-based, participatory framework (Wallerstein, 2002; Cheatham, 2003). The purpose was to gain the perspectives of youth participants and the adult leaders in order to develop program model guidelines for youth empowerment. Four community youth programs participated as research partners. The research processes included in-depth interviews with adult leaders, intensive on-site observations of the youth programs, youth engagement in a photo essay exercise, and adult and youth participation in a Youth Empowerment Program Summit.

# DIMENSIONS OF CRITICAL YOUTH EMPOWERMENT

Taken together, our examination of these four models and the results of our research with youth empowerment program, offer insights regarding six key dimensions of CYE:

- A welcoming and safe environment;
- Meaningful participation and engagement;
- Equitable power-sharing between youth and adults;
- Engagement in critical reflection on interpersonal and sociopolitical processes;
- Participation in sociopolitical processes to effect change; and
- Integrated individual- and community-level empowerment

Table 1 indicates which of these dimensions are highlighted across the four models, illustrating that each of the initial four models contains some of the dimensions in varying degrees, whereas the CYE model integrates all six. It is important to note the interrelated, dynamic nature of these six dimensions of CYE. In the following sections we examine each dimension in greater detail, discuss roles of adults and youth, and address potential challenges, opportunities, and benefits of the application of CYE in practice.

## A Welcoming and Safe Environment

A welcoming and safe social environment where youth feel valued, respected, encouraged, and supported is a key to CYE. Such an environment allows participants opportunities to share their feelings, take risks, and feel as if they belong to a family-like community (Heath, 1991). A welcoming and safe environment is a social space in which young people have freedom to be themselves, express their own creativity, voice their opinions in decision-making processes, try out new skills and roles, rise to challenges, and have fun in the process.

Environments conducive to CYE are those in which youth have a sense of ownership and yet are challenged and supported to move beyond their usual comfort zone; such environments are co-created by youth and adults. Although adults are often instrumental in bringing youth into programs and helping sustain their interest and participation, these activities and roles are not the exclusive domain of adults. For youth to fully participate and have ownership of the process, adults need to be able to ensure the necessary level of support, trust, and encourage-

TABLE 1. Dimensions of Critical Youth Empowerment Across the Models

| Dimensions | AEC | YDE | Transactional Partner | Empowering Education | Critical Youth Empowerment |
|---|---|---|---|---|---|
| Safe, supportive environment | Adults provide positive reinforcement. | **Adults, family support via high expectations, positive reinforcement.** | "Welcoming social climate" emphasized. | Supportive environment emphasized. | Environment must be safe, supportive, fun, caring, challenging. |
| Meaningful Participation | **Meaningful participation is critical for positive social bonding.** | Opportunity to learn skills, assume responsibility, participate in public affairs. | Structured process to develop and implement a youth-defined, community-based agenda | Structured experience includes interviewing, critically reflecting, and social action project. | Opportunities for youth to develop capacities in meaningful forum with youth responsibility and decision-making. |
| Shared Power | Shared power mentioned but not included in model. | Shared power mentioned but not included in model. | Incremental transfer of power to youth as they gain competence and confidence. | Adults and youths are co-learners; shared leadership discussed but not emphasized in model. | Shared power critical, incremental transfer of power to youth as they gain capacity. |
| Individual- and Community-level oriented | | Focused on individual-level development through participation in community affairs. | Individual- and community-level goals of esteem and capacity building. | Individual- and community-empowerment viewed as interwoven. | Individual- and community-empowerment viewed as interwoven. |
| Socio-political change goals | | Contribute to community affairs but not for goals of social change. | Contribute to community affairs but not for goals of social change. | Dialogue stage includes societal analysis and leads into social action projects. | Programs emphasize societal analysis and encourage social change goals. |
| Critical Reflection | Critical awareness mentioned but not demonstrated. | | Critical awareness and reflection mentioned but not demonstrated. | Dialogue stage includes societal analysis through structured questions. | Critical reflection integral to CYE through varied youth-based approaches. |

Bold: emphasized in model.
Plain: mentioned in article but not emphasized as a dimension of the model.
Blank: not mentioned in article.

ment, but retreat to the background so that youth can be the principal actors on what they perceive as center stage. Ideally, as Wallerstein et al. (2005) pointed out, youth and adults experience many opportunities to interact as co-learners.

From a CYE perspective, a welcoming safe environment is one in which youth have the opportunity to experience both success and failure. In the youth programs we observed, adults assumed the primary responsibility for ensuring the creation of the physical, social, emotional, and creative spaces where youth could explore and try out new skills, build personal and collective capacities, experience success, or make mistakes (Messias et al., 2005). A key role for adults is to ensure that failures do not lead to negative outcomes such as decreased self-esteem

or confidence (Cargo, 2003). Direct and indirect support, encouragement, and feedback from adults contribute to maintaining an environment conducive to youth actualization processes, especially when
activities or events fail. An important implication for CYE is that when
adults recognize that constructive learning can arise from failure as well
as success, they may need to monitor their own behaviors, presence, and
activities in order to let youth experience the consequences of their own
actions (Messias et al., 2005).

A supportive environment also includes promoting the positive potential and actual achievements of youth within the community (Kim,
1998; Cargo, 2003). Youth recognize that adults have power and the
value of using adult power to support their own causes. For example,
youth participants in our research commented that adult leaders could
provide "clout" for the youth and their community-based efforts in a society that is otherwise skeptical of the capabilities and intentions of
teenagers (Royce, 2004; Royce, April 2004).

## Meaningful Participation and Engagement

Opportunities to engage in meaningful activities through which
youth make an authentic contribution are essential to CYE efforts. Participation in community affairs provides opportunities for youth to learn
and practice important leadership and participatory skills (e.g., planning, organizing, oral and written communication) and try on different
roles and responsibilities. Youth need to engage in activities relevant to
their own lives, ones that excite and challenge them and "count as real"
(Heath, 1994, p. 289). Kim et al. (1998) stressed the notion that activities need to promote underlying competence and intrinsic motivations
of youth so that they can test and master their own interests, develop
skills, and gain confidence. Teen organizations often experience a high
turnover rate. Meaningful participation can contribute to more sustained and prolonged engagement, necessary for skill development and
mastery and positive youth identity development (Cargo, 2003).

Contributing to the larger community through authentic engagement
can help adolescents to combat rolelessness; in turn, meaningful roles
can provide youth with opportunities to develop a positive self-identity,
increased sense of self-worth, and enhanced self-efficacy (Chinman,
1998). Cargo et al. (2003, p. 577) argued that meaningful participation
includes facing and overcoming challenges:

Youth capacity was enhanced through healthful adaptation to those challenges associated with taking responsibility for their quality of life issues. Challenge is essential for human development as it allows people to actualize their potential as they respond and adapt to difficult situations.

Meaningful participation and engagement goes beyond simply "being present" at school or community-based activities. Engagement in community service and/or community change is only part of the process of meaningful participation. Wallerstein and colleagues (2005) demonstrated how in addressing health issues, youth were first actively engaged by interviewing, critically reflecting, and dialoguing about health issues, a process that prepared them to participate in community efforts with richer insights and capacity for action.

CYE emphasizes the need for authentic, youth-determined activities that challenge youth to engage in new roles and develop new skills and insights while also engaging in critical reflection and action. For youth to have meaningful experiences of leadership there must be varied opportunities to engage in, practice, and apply specific leadership skills. This includes having the responsibility for decision-making. Thus, meaningful participation is intricately enmeshed with another dimension of CYE, that of equitable power-sharing between youth and adults.

### Equitable Power-Sharing Between Youth and Adults

Several models addressed opportunities for youth to take on leadership roles (Chinman & Linney, 1998; Kim et al., 1998), which supports development of valuable leadership skills; however, many leadership roles in youth organizations come with little decision-making power, an additional factor important to consider. Power is a paradoxical, systemic phenomenon that permeates human functioning and interactions at multiple levels (Pinderhughes, 1995). In a society where adults hold legitimate power and are ultimately responsible for decisions and actions, creating equitable power-sharing within the contexts of youth empowerment programs is a challenge. For CYE to transpire, organizations need to examine attitudes, ideas, and activities related to power and power-sharing. In theory, youth-center power is associated with youth empowerment programs. However, in practice it is often difficult to achieve and maintain an equitable balance of decision-making and power within youth programs. Adults may believe that they are sharing power by assigning youth participants to committees. However, as Checkoway (1998) noted, agencies may favor such apparently safe methods because they tend to provide positive public relations and serve administrative ends. Yet such token participation rarely results in effective transfer of power to youth participants or real opportunities for youth to influence organizational decision-making.

Youth-determined and youth-directed activities are essential for CYE, but these rarely occur without some level of adult support and guidance. From a CYE perspective, a role of adult leaders is to create and maintain a balance of providing support without domination. In practice, this was observed as having high expectations for youth to take the lead, yet being available and providing guidance and support when needed. Such support is important if youth are to stretch to take on new responsibilities, try out new ideas, reach out into the community, and begin to make important decisions on behalf of the group.

Enacting shared leadership with youth takes commitment, effort, and insight about shared power. As described in the TP model, shared leadership may require considerable flexibility to effectively facilitate, teach, guide, mentor, encourage, provide feedback, keep youth focused and on task, yet exert authority and control when needed, without dominating and discouraging youth. In order to promote CYE, youth programs need to find ways of taking advantage of the experience and knowledge offered by adult leaders and structure the program in ways that enhance youth decision making and leadership.

Maintaining a delicate balance of overt support and covert control is a significant challenge for adults working towards CYE. We have noted considerable variation in the extent and visibility of adult power and control within youth programs. However, even in programs where the extent of adult power and control was not clearly visible, our participatory observations over time and in-depth interviews with adult leaders revealed ways in which they wielded power and control in each of the programs. Examples of strategies aimed at managing or controlling youth behaviors and activities included formal behavioral contracts, activity monitoring, and communication of specific program guidelines and expectations (Messias et al., 2005). We also observed a few seasoned adult leaders providing much support and guidance throughout a project and then fading into the background when it came to youths' public presentation, although this critical balance was difficult to achieve consistently.

One strategy for promoting CYE is for adults to transfer decision-making gradually over time (Cargo et al., 2003). In turn, youth need time and support to learn how to effectively harness power that they may have never had before (Zeldin, 2003). By creating opportunities for youth to develop competency in planning and implementation responsibilities, adults can then balance their role more towards an active enabler in planning an implementation "rather than being the 'well-intentioned practitioner' doing for youth" (Cargo, 2003, p. S70).

Our research suggested that shared power may come most readily in smaller, localized sites where youth are fully engaged in the local community and risks are lower than in larger organizations (Royce et al., 2004). For example, in the case of a state-wide diversity initiative, youth had more decision-making power in their school-based task force groups than they did at the state-level of the organization. Similarly, youth in a church-based anti-drug program had little effective decision-making power except in the context of a small improvisation theatre group, where participants made decisions about the content and style of their anti-drug skits. Smaller, localized efforts such as these may be a starting point for changing the fundamental structures of governance needed to support young people in leadership and decision-making roles.

Wheeler (2003) suggested that "each structural change addresses a fundamental shift in assumptions about adult privilege and youth responsibility, a shift that must occur in order for youth to participate genuinely in leadership and civic engagement" (p. 7). Structural formats that may need to be addressed or changed include modes of communication (i.e., adults tend to value the telephone whereas youth may rely more on email), executive leadership membership (i.e., including youth as full-fledged board members) and scheduling (i.e., inability of students to attend meetings due to time restrictions during the school day). Those with international experience in youth governance practices have suggested that such changes in structure will only come about when scholars and policy makers work with adult leaders to "persuade them of the benefits of a more open and democratic relationship with children and young people" (Lansdown, 2001; Zeldin, 2003, p. 13).

### Engagement in Critical Reflection on Interpersonal and Sociopolitical Processes

Critical empowerment involves multi-level processes through which individuals and communities become emancipated from conscious or unconscious constraints and engage in negotiated actions to build community life (Ray, 1992). If the goal of CYE is to transform people's lives and communities, inclusion of critical reflection in a youth empowerment effort is imperative. However, of the key dimensions of CYE, critical reflection is perhaps the one that has received less emphasis in practice. Of the four models we analyzed, only the EE model stressed development of critical awareness and reflection with a focus on social and political processes and structures. The other three models incorporated other processes of critical reflection and analysis to varying degrees. These included the need for increasing youths' understanding of community, institutional, and bureaucratic structures; participation in assessment of community resources; and reflecting on challenging events in order to form subsequent actions.

The relative lack of examples of socially transformative youth projects may be explained by the fact that, prior to engaging in effective sociopolitical action, critical reflection is required to help youth come to see and understand the very structures, processes, social values and practices that they seek to alter. As Freire (1970) argued, if people are not critically aware of the visible and invisible structures and processes that make up social institutions and practices, nor of their own role and actions within these institutions and practices, there is little room for empowerment. In this same tradition, Purdey, Adhikari, Robinson, and Cox (1994) argued that "capacity-building results from an ongoing and repetitive process of analysis, action, and reflection. The term *empowerment* is a reflexive verb, signifying that individuals can only empower themselves" (p. 330).

The development of social responsibility "requires critical thinking and ongoing support to maintain the commitment to work on problems over he long term, despite having an appreciation for the difficulties of both personal and social change" (Wallerstein et al., 2005, p. 229). Youth programs tend to focus on activities, leaving little time or space for reflection. Although reflecting on a program's activities is important, the challenge is to provide youth opportunities to engage in an integrated participatory cycle of critical reflection and reflective actions with the goal of creating change in sociopolitical processes, structures, norms, and images. This type of critical reflection requires time, space, and commitment. It also requires adult leaders who are attuned to the sociopolitical realities of the topic at hand, and who have the skills and knowledge needed to guide youth in such critical examinations. For example, in the EE projects, the researchers were integrally involved in the design and day-to-day activities of the youth empowerment program. They provided ongoing training and supervision to adult facilitators (graduate and undergraduate students who earned course credit) in guiding youth through critical reflection activities through which young people sought deeper understandings of the social and political processes that underlie addiction (Wallerstein, 1999).

Youth-centered opportunities for guided reflection and discussion can be both enjoyable and intellectually challenging (DiBenedetto, 1992). In addition to developing skills in facilitating critical reflection, adult leaders need to consider methods that appeal to young people. Photography, music, theater, and graphic arts can serve as triggers for reflection as well as the medium through which youth can express their views and messages regarding social issues (Messias et al., 2005).

## Participation in Sociopolitical Processes in Order to Effect Change

Essential to CYE is the notion that youth participation within the community includes engagement in sociopolitical processes and social change. This does not exclude youth participation in civic service, but rather incorporates social change efforts within such service. For example, youth serving as reading tutors might organize around issues of poverty and literacy, seeking to address structures and processes that result in illiteracy in low income communities and the need for tutors in the first place. The difference between civic service and critical social engagement distinguishes CYE from youth development, which emphasizes helping "adolescents become competent, engaged, and responsible adults" (Roth, 1998, p. 423). From a CYE perspective, youth are not truly empowered if they do not have the capacity to address the structures, processes, social values and practices of the issues at hand. As Zimmerman (1995) argued, empowerment is about gaining mastery within a given social environment. Such mastery entails understanding the underlying processes and practices of that environment and how to best influence them.

CYE involves youth gaining a critical understanding of the underlying processes and mastery through participation in transformative social action. In both the EE and TP models, youth empowerment was envisioned as occurring through participation in social actions. However, the notion is not necessarily fully realized in community practice with youth. Wallerstein and colleagues (1994, 2005) described several community action projects that seek to change policy (e.g., youth recommendations to their tribal council to address alcohol-related problems) or to critically educate the broader public about an issue through student-developed films or plays. However, other projects based on the EE model, such as developing a youth center or becoming peer educators, while important and worthwhile actions, were not representative of actions that result in systemic change.

Although transformative engagement is difficult to locate in adult-sponsored youth organizations, there is a growing body of research is beginning to document the potential for youth to contribute to social change. For example, participants in the Long Beach Health Opportunities, Problem-Solving, and Empowerment (HOPE) project for Asian American girls received leadership training that involved researching a social issue of their choice in their local community. The resulting policy recommendations for addressing sexual harassment were implemented throughout the school district (Cheatham, 2003). In a summary report, Zeldin et al. (2003) provided examples in which youth engagement in community action benefited the youth and the community, leading to increased resources and opportunities, and a community more responsive to the needs of a diverse public. Our research with youth organizations exemplified empowerment that can arise from effecting change of social images, values, and norms. In the process of developing photo essays on the theme "how youth make a difference in the community," some of the youth participants purposefully addressed specific community actions to counter negative societal images of youth.

## *Integrated Individual and Community-Level Empowerment*

Critical youth empowerment integrates opportunities and results in positive change at both individual and community levels. Programs that empower youth need to provide opportunities for development at both individual and community levels. All four models illustrated the value of providing individual youth with opportunities for personal development through learning and applying valuable skills for navigating adult worlds, thereby increasing self-efficacy. It is also important that youth experience opportunities for engagement with diverse sectors within the local community. As Zimmerman (2000) noted, empowering processes at the community level include access to resources, tolerance for diversity, and open governance structures. Many youth empowerment programs offer civic service opportunities for youth that provide them with stronger ties to the community, a greater understanding of other people's needs, and a commitment to making that community a better place. Such opportunities can promote collective- and political-efficacy in addition to self-efficacy.

Furthermore, the community is improved when a more diverse representation of citizens is engaged in building civil society. Integrated community-level outcomes include effective and active organizational coalitions, pluralistic leadership, and increased participatory skills among individual community members. For example, Zeldin et al. (2003) found that youth engagement in community organizations produced "ripple effects" throughout the community. As some of the organizations gained visibility through their youth engagement and community outreach efforts, they established new standards for other organizations and local foundations. Cargo et al. (2003) described a similar progression of social integration that ultimately results in social bonding, a progression predicted by the YD&E model. Once youth gained access to traditionally adult-run committees, over time there was a shift in community norms toward an expectation that youth would sit on the committees.

Critical social empowerment involves both individual and group level change: enhancing the capacity of individuals to contribute to and work in collaboration with others to effect social change. It is important to recognize the capacity of youth to contribute to the benefit of the communities within which they live–school, neighborhood, city, state, and even national and global communities (Zeldin et al., 2003). However, if being empowered means having agency, then youth need to develop a critical awareness of processes, structures, social practices, norms, and images that affect them, so that they can determine how to live productively within those social spaces or, better yet, how to change them for the benefit of all. As evident in Rissel's (1994) work, most definitions of critical change focus upon changing policies and institutional structures. A CYE framework envisions the capacity for change to organizational, institutional, and societal policies, structures, processes, social values, norms, and images.

From the perspective of critical social theories, youth empowerment is not complete without critical reflection, reflective action, and social change at individual and collective levels. Youth may be able to address community problems, but if they do not have opportunities to examine the sociopolitical processes that underpin and created these community problems, then they lack the insight needed to become effective agents for altering the status quo (e.g., Freire, 1970). For example, youth might determine that too many teens smoke, leading them to develop a campaign to reduce smoking among their peers. However, such actions do not lead youth to understand the sociopolitical forces that encourage teen smoking, such as marketing strategies by tobacco companies that target youth, nor do these actions lead youth to develop the requisite skills and knowledge for altering the sociopolitical forces.

One particular challenge for CYE is effectively integrating individual, community, and political empowerment among groups of low-income and minority youths. Formation of community partnerships is one approach that has led to successful programs in establishing networks among community agencies which serve high-risk populations (Kim et al., 1998). Focusing these efforts on sociopolitical issues would enhance CYE.

## Benefits and Outcomes

When these six dimensions are fully integrated within youth programs, there are numerous potential benefits to youth and communities. Individual-level developmental outcomes for youth include increased self-efficacy and self-awareness as well as positive identity development, positive social bonding, awareness of organizational operations and interpersonal relations, and a sense of purpose (Cargo et al., 2003; Chinman & Linney, 1998; Kim et al., 1998; Wallerstein et al., 2005). Inter-personal outcomes include opportunities for adults and youth to spend time together, recognize each other's strengths and assets, and value partnership and collaboration, thereby bridging existing divides and further integrating young people into larger social worlds (Chinman & Linney, 1998; Kim et al., 1998). Community engagement provides benefits of social integration and expansion of life chances and social networks and also enhances participatory competence, such as the capacity to cooperation, compromise, and appreciate diverse perspectives (Cargo et al., 2003).

Finally, there are several outcomes of community-level empowerment. CYE promotes self-, collective-, and political-efficacy through youth-led community engagements that focus on sociopolitical change (Wallerstein et al., 2005). From a CYE perspective, youth are not truly empowered if they do not have the capacity to address the structures, processes, social values and practices of the issues at hand. Socially integrating youth in responsible roles with shared power encourages community development that better serves not only the needs of youth, but potentially the needs of all community members (Zeldin et al., 2003). CYE potentially benefits youth and community in numerous ways, through empowering processes that lead to both individual- and community-level empowerment. Assessment and measurement of these outcomes and processes is one of the challenges of youth empowerment programs.

### Measuring Critical Youth Empowerment

In evaluating the impact and outcomes of youth empowerment programs, it is useful to make the distinction between empowerment as a process and an outcome. An empowering process is a series of experiences where youth, adults, organizations and communities engage in collective action for social change. The six dimensions described here provide a frame of reference for creating these opportunities for youth and can also guide evaluation efforts. It is important to note that empowering processes occur at multiple levels (individual, organizations, community) and each level will have related outcomes. This is complicated by the fact that empowerment is not experienced in the same way by individuals, organizations and communities. Therefore, the development of a global measure of empowerment is not an appropriate goal (Zimmerman, 2000). In the arena of youth empowerment research, measurement of psychological empowerment is a fairly well developed area. However, progress in assessment of community outcomes presents more complex methodological challenges, such as multi-method triangulation. However, addressing community evaluation as a participatory process in which youth are actively engaged in the design, implementation, and analysis of evaluation studies should be considered an opportunity for meaningful engagement and empowerment. As such, empowerment evaluation is a promising area for future community-based, youth-centered research.

## IMPLICATIONS FOR FUTURE RESEARCH AND PRACTICE

This examination of existing models of youth empowerment has laid the groundwork for an expanded, integrated theory of youth empowerment from a critical social perspective. Yet further conceptualization and research is needed on the multiple, complex processes and the intergenerational nature and sociopolitical change goals of CYE.

A major practice implication is the need for education and training of adults with the aim of increasing conscious power-sharing, guiding youth and adults through critical reflection activities, and supporting the broad goal of critical social youth empowerment. It has been suggested that youth and adults would benefit from training that focuses on building youth-adult partnerships (Sherrod, 2002), although existing models of youth empowerment have not provided details about how to support adults in developing this balance. Research is needed to examine and illustrate processes of supporting adult leaders in striking a balance between guiding and directing (Zeldin et al., 2003).

Further practice-based research is needed to further understand how engagement in CYE may influence youth differentially. Individual youth, youth groups, and communities, will not experience empowerment in the same way. The intersections of other potential power inequalities and differentials (e.g., race, class, gender, culture, language, immigration status, sexuality) are another area for further examination within the CYE framework. Development and evaluation of effective community-based practice and research is a promising and critical opportunity to further the goal of CYE to promote participatory processes in which adults and youth work collectively to change the status quo toward more equitable, just, healthy processes, practices, structures, images and social values.

# REFERENCES

Campbell, J. B., S. (1991). "Voices and paradigms: Perspectives on critical and feminist theory in nursing." *Advances in Nursing Science, 13*, 1-15.

Cargo, M., Grams, G.D., Ottoson, J. M., Ward, P., & Green, L.W. (2003). "Empowerment as fostering positive youth development and citizenship." *American Journal of Health Behavior, 27*(Supplement 1), S66-79.

Cheatham, A., & Shen, E. (2003). Community based participatory research with Cambodian girls in Long Beach, California: A case study. In M. M. N. Wallerstein (Ed.), *Community based participatory research for health* (pp. 316-331). San Francisco: John Wiley & Sons Inc./Jossey Bass.

Checkoway, B. (1998). Involving young people in neighborhood development. *Children & Youth Services Review, 20*(9), 765-795.

Chinman, M. J., & Linney, J.A. (1998). Toward a model of adolescent empowerment: Theoretical and empirical evidence. *Journal of Primary Prevention, 18*, 393-413.

DiBenedetto, A. (1992). Youth groups: A model for empowerment. *Networking Bulletin* 2(3): 19-24.

Freire, P. (1970). *The pedagogy of the oppressed*. New York: Seabury Press.

Heath, S. B., & McLaughlin, M.W. (1991). Community organizations as family–Endeavors that engage and support adolescents. *Phi Delta Kappan, 72*(8), 623-627.

Heath, S. B., & McLaughlin, M.W. (1994). The best of both worlds: Connecting schools and community youth organizations for all-day, all-year learning. *Educational Administration Quarterly, 30*(3), 278-300.

Jennings, L.B., & Green, J.L. (1999). Locating democratizing and transformative practices within classroom discourse. *Journal of Classroom Interaction, 34*(2), i-iv.

Jones, P. S., & Meleis, A. I. (1993). Health is empowerment. *Advances in Nursing Science, 15*(3), 1-14.

Kim, S., Crutchfield, C., Williams, C., & Hepler, N. (1998). Toward a new paradigm in substance abuse and other problem behavior prevention for youth: Youth development and empowerment approach. *Journal of Drug Education, 28*(1), 1-17.

Lansdown, G. (2001). *Promoting children's participation in democratic decision-making.* UNICEF Innocenti Research Center, Florence, Italy.

Messias, D. K. H., Fore, M.E., McLoughlin, K., & Parra-Medina, D. (2005). Adults roles in community-based youth empowerment programs: Implications for best practices. *Family & Community Health, 28*(4), 320-337.

Pinderhughes, E. (1995). Empowering diverse populations: Family practices in the 21st century. *Families in Society, 76*(3), 131-140.

Purdey, A.F., Adhikari, G.B., Robinson, S.A., & Cox, P.W. (1994). Participatory health development in rural Nepal: Clarifying the process of community empowerment. *Health Education Quarterly, 21*(3), 329-343.

Rappaport, J. (1984). Studies in empowerment: Introduction to the issue. *Prevention in Human Services, 3*, 1-7.

Rappaport, J. (1987). Terms of empowerment/exemplars of prevention: Toward a theory for community psychology. *American Journal of Community Psychology, 15*(2), 121-148.

Ray, M. A. (1992). Critical theory as a framework to enhance nursing science. *Nursing Science Quarterly, 5*(3), 98-101.

Rissel, C. (1994). Empowerment–The holy grail of health promotion. *Health Promotion International, 9*(1), 39-47.

Rocha, E.M. (1997). A ladder of empowerment. *Journal of the American Planning Association, 17*, 31-44.

Roth, J., Brooks-Gunn, J., Murray, L., & Foster, W. (1998). Promoting healthy adolescents: Synthesis of youth development program evaluations. *Journal of Research on Adolescence, 8*(4), 423-459.

Royce, S. (2004). *Hearing their voices: Using Photovoice to capture youth perspectives on empowerment.* Columbia, University of South Carolina.

Royce, S., Jennings, L. B., & McLaughlin, K. (2004, April). *Youth Perspectives on Youth Empowerment: Informing Theory and Practice.* Paper presented at the American Educational Research Association Annual Meeting, San Diego, CA.

Sherrod, L., Flannagan, C.L., & Youniss, J. (2002). Dimensions of citizenship and opportunities for youth development: The what, when, why, where and who of citizenship development. *Applied Development Science, 6*, 264-272.

Small, S., & Memmo, M. (2004). Contemporary models of youth development and problem prevention: Toward an integration of terms, concepts, and models. *Family Relations, 53*, 3-11.

Wallerstein, N. (1992). Powerlessness, empowerment, and health: Implications for health promotion programs. *American Journal of Health Promotion, 6*(3), 197-205.

Wallerstein, N., & Bernstein, E. (1988). Empowerment Education–Freire Ideas Adapted to Health-Education. *Health Education Quarterly, 15*(4), 379-394.

Wallerstein, N., & Duran, B. (2002). The conceptual, historical, and practice roots of community based participatory research and related participatory traditions. In M.

Minkler & N. Wallerstein (Eds.), *Community-Based Participatory Research for Health* (pp. 27-52). San Francisco: Jossey-Bass.

Wallerstein, N., & Sanchez-Merki, V. (1994). Freirian-praxis in health-education research: Results from an adolescent prevention program. *Health Education Resources, 9*(1), 105-118.

Wallerstein, N., Sanchez-Merki, V., & Dow, L. (1999). Freirian praxis in health education and community organizing: A case study of an adolescent prevention program. In M. Minkler (Ed.), *Community organizing and community building for health.* New Brunswick: Rutgers University Press.

Wallerstein, N., Sanchez-Merki, V., & Verlade, L. (2005). Freirian praxis in health education and community organizing: A case study of an adolescent prevention program. In M. Minkler (Ed.), *Community Organizing and Community Building for Health, 2nd ed.* New Brunswick, NJ: Rutgers University Press.

Wheeler, W. (2003) Creating structural change to support youth development. *Social Policy Report: Giving Child and Youth Development Knowledge Away, 17*(3), p. 7.

Zeldin, S., Camino, L., & Calvert, M. (2003). Toward an understanding of youth in community governance: Policy priorities and research directions. *Social Policy Report: Giving Child and Youth Development Knowledge Away, 17*(3), 1-20.

Zimmerman, M. A. (1995). Psychological empowerment: Issues and illustrations. *American Journal of Community Psychology, 23*(5), 581-599.

Zimmerman, M. A. (2000). Empowerment theory: Psychological, organizational, and community levels of analysis. In J. R. E. Seidmann (Ed.), *Handbook of community psychology.* New York: Kluwer Academic/Plenum.

Zimmerman, M. A., & Rappaport, J. (1988). Citizen participation, perceived control, and psychological empowerment. *American Journal of Community Psychology, 16*(5), 725-750.

# Sariling Gawa Youth Council as a Case Study of Youth Leadership Development in Hawai'i

Esminia M. Luluquisen, DrPH, MPH, RN
Alma M. O. Trinidad, MSW
Dipankar Ghosh, DO

**SUMMARY.** This article describes *Sariling Gawa* Youth Council as a case study of youth leadership development in Hawai'i. Since 1980, thousands of young people–primarily Filipino youth–have participated in *Sariling Gawa* activities which have developed their leadership skills. Many of them have continued to lead the organization and utilize what they learned with numerous local organizations and state agencies. The authors examine *Sariling Gawa*'s growth, structure, and other factors that contribute to its longevity. The model includes (1) youth empowerment through building their leadership skills, (2) fostering and strengthening peer social support and social networks, (3) promotion of positive

Esminia M. Luluquisen is Adjunct Faculty, San Francisco State University, Department of Community Health Education. Alma M. O. Trinidad is a PhD student, University of Washington, School of Social Work. Dipankar Ghosh is Resident Physician, Alameda County Medical Center.

Address correspondence to: Esminia M. Luluquisen, DrPH, 1600 Holloway Avenue-HSS 204, San Francisco, CA 94132-4161 (E-mail: emluluq@sfsu.edu).

[Haworth co-indexing entry note]: "*Sariling Gawa* Youth Council as a Case Study of Youth Leadership Development in Hawai'i." Luluquisen, Esminia M., Alma M. O. Trinidad, and Dipankar Ghosh. Co-published simultaneously in *Journal of Community Practice* (The Haworth Press, Inc.) Vol. 14, No. 1/2, 2006, pp. 57-70; and: *Youth Participation and Community Change* (ed: Barry N. Checkoway, and Lorraine M. Gutiérrez) The Haworth Press, Inc., 2006, pp. 57-70. Single or multiple copies of this article are available for a fee from The Haworth Document Delivery Service [1-800-HAWORTH, 9:00 a.m. - 5:00 p.m. (EST). E-mail address: docdelivery@haworthpress.com].

ethnic identity, and (4) community capacity building by involving youth in civic and community affairs. *[Article copies available for a fee from The Haworth Document Delivery Service: 1-800-HAWORTH. E-mail address: <docdelivery@haworthpress.com> Website: <http://www.HaworthPress.com> © 2006 by The Haworth Press, Inc. All rights reserved.]*

**KEYWORDS.** Filipino youth, immigrant youth, youth leadership development, youth-led organizations

## DEVELOPMENT IN HAWAI'I

For the past twenty-five years, *Sariling Gawa* Youth Council, Inc. (*Sariling Gawa*) has been conducting a youth leadership development program, led by college age youth and young adults in Hawai'i. *Sariling Gawa* started as a grassroots community effort in 1980, within the context of commemorating Filipinos' historical roots in Hawai'i. The significance of this quarter of a century effort is that social service, education and public health professionals working in agencies did not create the organization. Instead, a group of college students began the organization by reflecting, analyzing and acting on their experiences of being immigrant, Filipino and young in Hawai'i. Since its inception, thousands of young people have participated in *Sariling Gawa* activities to develop their leadership skills; many continued to utilize what they learned in their work with numerous local and state agencies and organizations. Interestingly, the majority of *Sariling Gawa* past and current board members, planners, mentors and trainers were former youth leaders. *Sariling Gawa* has become an example of a community-wide intervention that builds youth leaders and fosters pro-social social norms among youth.

Filipinos comprise a large segment of people in Hawai'i at 14.1% of the total state's population in the 2000 U.S. Census. In the United States, Filipinos comprise the second largest Asian population after the Chinese (U.S. Census Bureau, 2000). In the 1980s, Filipino community members in Hawai'i were concerned over a comparatively low educational attainment of the youth and an increasing gang involvement (Asuncion, Domingo, Macugay, Saludes-Galvez, & Los Banos, 1981). Recent studies on Filipino youth in Hawai'i indicate that they encounter numerous adverse health and behavioral outcomes. For example, middle school Filipino children had a higher rate of making plans to kill themselves compared to the general middle school rate (Centers for Disease Control & Prevention, 2002). Filipino adolescents in Hawai'i have a high lifetime and daily prevalence of tobacco, any cigarettes, and alcohol (Pearson & Oliveira, 2002). With regards to alcohol, the lifetime prevalence rate for alcohol among Filipino 6th graders in 2000 was higher than the state's rate (Pearson & Oliveira, 2002). Among all ethnic groups in Hawai'i, Filipino youth comprise the highest percentage of gang membership (Chesney-Lind et al., 1992; Chesney-Lind et al., 1995). In 2003, Filipinos came in third following Native Hawaiian and White in all arrests for juveniles (Gao & Perrone, 2004).

This article explores how *Sariling Gawa* has contributed to ensuring that Filipino youth have the support and opportunities to realize their maximum potential for personal growth, civic engagement and community participation. The paper first describes *Sariling Gawa*'s growth and evolution and its organizational structure, to provide insight into its longevity and sustainability. The next section examines its youth leadership development model against research literature on the ecological factors that affect the health outcomes of youth. A case study approach is used, utilizing data from document reviews, key informant interviews, focus groups and participant observation (Yin, 1993; Yin, 1994; Stake, 1994; Stake, 1995).

## *SARILING GAWA'S GROWTH AND EVOLUTION*

Go to the people
Live among them
Learn from them
Start with what they know
Build on what they have.
But the best leaders
When their task is accomplished
Their work is done
The people all remark
'We have done it ourselves.'

Anonymous

From the beginning, the above poem has described the organization's mission (Asuncion et al., 1981). The college students who created *Sariling Gawa* adopted the values underlying the poem to promote and institutionalize, among Filipino youth throughout the state of Hawai'i, their involvement, cooperation and leadership within every aspect of the organization. These same college students believed that a youth leadership program needed to cultivate teamwork as they addressed issues that most affected them. *Sariling Gawa* was thus chosen as the name, translated from *Tagalog* (a Filipino language) to mean "our own work" (Asuncion et al., 1981). Moreover, they asserted: "through community involvement and ongoing education, *Sariling Gawa* will increase the number of well-informed Filipino leaders as well as ordinary citizens who will contribute to the growth of the community" (Asuncion et al., 1981).

Over the years, *Sariling Gawa* has undergone three distinct stages of growth during its twenty-five years of existence: creation, expansion and sustainability. In the creation phase, roughly the first five years of the organization's existence, the original group of founders worked to establish an organization with a strong identity and a capable leadership body. The founders also wanted to establish a symbol for the organization that had roots in the Filipino culture and traditions. *Sariling Gawa*'s logo was formulated to be that of a growing coconut sprout because it "represents the Filipino youth being nurtured by the older, more established Filipino community in Hawai'i as symbolized by the mature coconut. The coconut plant is adaptable to any tropical setting throughout the world just as the Filipinos have adapted to Hawai'i. . . . When a coconut washes ashore and gives birth to a sprout, it develops deep roots . . . (that) are strong enough to withstand hurricanes and high waves in much the same way the Filipinos have established strong roots in Hawai'i and have experienced strong struggles against discrimination in employment, education, housing, and government" (Asuncion et al., 1981, p. ii).

The youth who were involved during this phase debated over the mission, goals, and direction of the organization and worked out their differences and conflicts. Several adult leaders of the community, predominantly professors from the University of Hawai'i and educators in the school system, provided the fledgling group with the necessary resources. Under the tutelage of these mentors, this initial group of young people was able to establish a foundation for a sustainable project. The youth leaders utilized their skills to lead groups and conduct group process, take charge of program committees, offer public presentations, develop training curricula, plan and conduct conferences, and fundraise to offset some of the expenses to conduct the various activities (Asuncion et al., 1981).

During the expansion phase, lasting approximately ten years, subsequent groups of Filipino young people, primarily college students from the University of Hawai'i campuses, sustained and broadened the early efforts of the founding group. As members of various college-based clubs, they organized intercollegiate picnics, parties, celebrations, meetings and cultural events to strengthen bonds among Filipino youth. These gatherings were also used as the channels for attracting future *Sariling Gawa* participants and leaders. Moreover, university professors taught various courses in Ethnic Studies, Philippine Studies and Community Studies and provided their students with a field studies option through *Sariling Gawa*.

During the expansion phase, approximately one hundred new leaders joined *Sariling Gawa* among Filipino college students. Leaderships cohorts formed that continued the tradition of mentoring and training their successors. They also expanded the initial curriculum and improved upon the earlier efforts. Many of the young people returned year after year to volunteer, to lead groups, to serve on committees and/or the Board of Directors.

The current stage of "sustainability" is the result of having established a core of leaders who are dedicated to the organization and a core set of activities that Filipino youth are committed to conducting annually. Youth leaders have stated: "*Sariling Gawa* will live on forever" (Luluquisen, 2001). *Sariling Gawa* is a well-known youth organization in Hawai'i whereby the major Filipino community and college student groups and organizations such as the YMCA have a working relationship with members of the organization.

*Sariling Gawa* has three program components. Primarily, the program provides opportunities for youth leadership development for college students and young adults that involve training in directing a non-profit organization, leading groups, peer mentoring, role modeling and community mobilization. The second component involves youth development with an emphasis on building necessary social and learning skills, a positive and self-assured Filipino identity and participation in Filipino culture and community. Its third component is *Sariling Gawa*'s partnerships with other Filipino community organizations to provide avenues for Filipino youth to partake in various projects and cultural events, such as the Centennial Anniversary of Philippine Independence (Luluquisen, 2001).

*Sariling Gawa* strives to be egalitarian and cooperative in its organizational structure. Youth members as leaders share responsibilities to fulfill its original purpose that is embodied in the name "Our Own Work." Despite the existence of a more formal structure for over a decade, the predominant nature of the organization is one of shared leadership and shared workloads, thus utilizing the Filipino essence of a *barangay* (village, community, town governed by rules and values). In the 2004-2005 strategic planning sessions, *Sariling Gawa* youth and adult leaders reinforced the principles of cooperation and partnerships as they established a comprehensive program plan for the next five years.

Since its inception, core groups of youth have formed the leadership body to perform the majority of the organizational and programmatic tasks. The organization's main activity is to conduct the annual statewide leadership conference for Filipino youth, requiring teams of leaders to be responsible for all planning, recruitment, fundraising and operating the full conference. The organization's leaders are volunteers who are young college students, working young adults and adults. A program committee has the responsibility to develop the conference curriculum, conduct the leadership training sessions for conference leaders, promote *Sariling Gawa*, and recruit youths to register for the conference. This committee also works closely with the Board of Directors and with other Filipino organizations that serve as co-sponsors. Youth conference leaders are college students from Oahu's universities enrolled in a Philippine Studies or Ethnic Studies class. For course credit, they volunteer in a Filipino community activity, such as *Sariling Gawa*.

The organization's curriculum and activities promote a strong sense of cooperative learning aimed at increasing social, emotional, cognitive, behavioral, and moral competencies. Two groups of youth participate in *Sariling Gawa* activities: college students and high school students. The trainers have been previous conference leaders, under the age of 27, who participated in leadership training sessions. They have the responsibility to be facilitators and mentors for new youth leaders. Youth leaders are trained in leadership, communication, life and social skills, and personal development incorporating positive Filipino ethnic identity. After extensive training, youth leaders work together in teams to lead small groups (*barangays*). It is through small groups that participants learn from each other and where critical thinking and consciousness-raising occurs.

## ELEMENTS AND RATIONALE FOR SARILING GAWA'S YOUTH LEADERSHIP DEVELOPMENT MODEL

This section reviews *Sariling Gawa*'s four elements of youth leadership development: (1) youth empowerment through building their leadership skills; (2) fostering and strengthening peer social support and social networks among Filipino young people; (3) promoting positive ethnic identity; and (4) building community capacity by involving youth in civic, cultural, social, and community affairs. Findings from documents review, focus groups, and surveys provide the description of these elements. Research literature is also reviewed for the significance of the various elements related to promoting community and adolescent health.

## Youth Empowerment

Empowerment strives to achieve social change, both personally and politically, to meet human needs and elevate issues not readily addressed (Gutiérrez, Parsons, & Cox, 1998). Implicit in *Sariling Gawa*'s model is the essence of youth empowerment by focusing its strengths through teaching youth leadership skills relevant to the history, culture and socio-economic context of Filipinos in Hawai'i. *Sariling Gawa* began this youth leadership development focus from the start. During 1980-1985, the college student founders of *Sariling Gawa* received invaluable training on youth leadership from two master teachers with expertise in human development, group facilitation, conflict resolution and youth leadership. The founders subsequently recruited other young adult trainers to fortify the skills gained by *Sariling Gawa*'s fledgling cohort of youth leaders. The outcome of this early strategy was an annual leadership training *program* which has lasted for the past twenty-five years, whereby experienced youth leaders trained newer leaders to conduct a *Sariling Gawa* state-wide youth conference.

The current eight-week youth leadership training program covers topics in communication, decision-making, group facilitation skills, cultural and ethnic identity, Filipino history, and youth development. In each respective year from 2001 through 2005, an average of twenty youth and young adult trainers conducted interactive sessions with fifty college students. These sessions taught individual leadership skills necessary to lead a small group of high school youth that attend the annual statewide conferences.

Data gathered from group discussions with youth leaders and key informant interviews indicates that youth leaders gained skills in four main areas, as seen in Table 1. Moreover, *Sariling Gawa* has institutionalized mechanisms for Filipino youth to apply leadership skills with their peers and younger high school students. Youth take on a variety of leadership roles in operating the organization, coordinating events and

TABLE 1. Skills Learned by *Sariling Gawa* Leaders

| Life and social skills | Leadership skills |
|---|---|
| • how to access resources related to school, employment, health concerns (HIV/AIDS, sexuality, contraception, substance abuse)<br>• how to interact with youth and adults who are different than themselves<br>• understanding family dynamics and how to handle difficult situations with family and friends | • problem solving<br>• how to lead small and large groups<br>• how to organize youth<br>• how to plan, strategize and develop action plans<br>• how to promote team building in a group process |
| **Communication skills** | **Identity and personal development** |
| • how to ask questions<br>• how to speak in front of groups<br>• how to speak about problems<br>• how to give information and advice to other youth | • how to accept and be proud of Filipino ethnicity<br>• how to recognize the prejudice against Filipino immigrants and to counter it<br>• how to be proud of, learn and maintain Filipino language skills |

conferences and developing and implementing training programs (see Table 1. Skills Learned by *Sariling Gawa* Leaders).

## Peer Social Support and Community-Level Social Networks

*Sariling Gawa*'s application of peer social support and its efforts to strengthen the social network systems among Filipino youth are congruous with literature on the protective and buffering nature of social support networks (Berkman & Syme, 1979; DuBois, Felner, Brand, Adan, & Evans, 1992; Kuo & Tsai, 1986; Levitt & Levitt, 1994). Group social support is an integral component of *Sariling Gawa*'s youth leadership development model. The model provides ongoing opportunities and "meeting grounds" for social support networks to form among Filipino young people, including a sprinkling of youth from other ethnic groups across the state of Hawai'i.

The Filipino youth who have participated in *Sariling Gawa*'s youth leadership development program have also established extensive social networks in an effort to sustain mutual affective and material social support. They have created a structure for ongoing social interactions and linkages through which they reciprocate sharing resources, friendships, as well as personal, educational and business connections. Many *Sariling Gawa* participants have, in the long-term, expanded their relationships by becoming business partners, forming filial family relationships, or developing romantic partnerships that progressed into marriages (Luluquisen, 2001). These social networks have also functioned to validate each other's ethnic and social identity, to integrate network members into a set of social norms through the affirmation of what are appropriate behaviors and values and to help each other mobilize psychological resources when faced with emotional difficulties.

In addition to hosting informal gatherings and social activities, *Sariling Gawa* partners with public and private agencies, such as the YMCA, University of Hawai'i, and the United Filipino Council of Hawai'i, so that youth can engage in civic and community service projects throughout the state. For example, *Sariling Gawa* was integral to the planning and development of the Filipino Community Center that provides social services to the community and is currently involved with the 2005-2006 Filipino Centennial Commission's activities. Additionally, youth leaders have taken their skills to become directors, planners, counselors, attorneys and teachers in key agency positions.

There is apparent community collective efficacy and social capital among the Filipino youth leaders and participants that has also expanded into the larger community. *Sariling Gawa* leaders have established social networks to promote social change in the educational, social and civic sectors of the Hawai'i community. There is also evidence of the group's social capital. That is, the presence of trusting relationships among group members, whereby people feel connected, trusting and cooperative with others, promotes a sense of belonging and allows collective action (Easterling, Gallagher, & Johnson, 1998).

### Promoting Positive Ethnic Identity

Achieving a positive ethnic identity is an important milestone for all youth (Erikson, 1968; Phinney & Rosenthal, 1992). Youth of color and immigrant youth, however, face additional difficulties of dealing with racism and discrimination in this process. Negative effects of experiencing racism, prejudice, and discrimination may include personal feelings of worthlessness and shame. Youth may also deny membership within their own group and thus lose valuable social networks and support. Moreover, research has shown that youth who have experienced racism may achieve less in school, have lower aspirations for the future, and drop out of school in increased numbers (National Research Council, 2002; Parks, 1999; Utsey, Ponterotto, Reynolds & Cancelli, 2000).

Results from surveys conducted with *Sariling Gawa* participants in 1994, 1995 and 1996 revealed that they live in a social environment in which Filipinos and other ethnic groups experience varying levels of derogation. As a consequence of their negative experiences related to being Filipino, they did not want to claim their ethnicity, let alone know about it. The negative stereotypes produced in many of the Filipino youth feelings of shame of being Filipino or associating with persons that "look" Filipino. Moreover, "Filipino jokes" that they had heard repeatedly throughout their lives negatively affected their sense of ethnic identity (Luluquisen, 2001).

Accordingly, *Sariling Gawa*'s youth leadership development program addresses ethnic identity development. The program teaches skills that include (1) how to accept and be proud of ethnicity despite experiencing racism and discrimination, (2) how to recognize the prejudice against Filipino immigrants and to counter it, especially with other Filipino youth and (3) how to learn, maintain and be proud of Filipino language skills.

A strong focus on developing a positive ethnic identity has resonated well with youth leaders. Recent youth immigrants from the Philippines stated that they have been attracted to *Sariling Gawa* because of their desire and need to have friends who are similar to them, ethnically and culturally. These recently immigrated youths must learn how to acculturate into another society while maintaining deeply held Filipino traditions. Their participation in *Sariling Gawa* has provided them with a familiar cultural context as they are transitioning into American culture and society. Among Filipino youth who experienced being teased, derogated and physically attacked for being Filipino, *Sariling Gawa* has provided the opportunity to learn and express their culture among peers who recognize the value of their ethnic heritage (Luluquisen, 2001).

### Community Capacity Building

*Sariling Gawa* was created to strengthen the Filipino community's social, economic and educational well-being through fostering youth leadership. Easterling et al. (1998) noted five elements of community capacity building that are incorporated into S*ariling Gawa's* efforts: (1) skills and knowledge that allow for more effective actions and programs; (2) leadership that allows a community to draw together and take advantage of the various talents and skills that are present among its members; (3) a sense of efficacy and confidence that encourages community members to step forward and take the sorts of actions that will enhance the community's well-being; (4) trusting relationships among members that promote collective problem-solving and reciprocal care-giving (social capital); and (5) a culture of learning that allows its members to feel comfortable exploring new ideas and learning from their experience.

Numerous youth who participated in the *Sariling Gawa*'s leadership development program became leaders in a variety of Filipino civic and community organizations. They attributed their desire to be leaders in multiple arenas to the skills and confidence gained from *Sariling Gawa*. Youth leaders have engaged in school based Filipino clubs, community organizations, Hawai'i statewide committees and cultural events, such as the 2005-2006 Filipino Centennial Celebration Commission. Moreover, youth leaders have not limited their engagement to Filipino community groups but have expanded their activities to organizations such as the Hawai'i State Nursing Association, the National Association of Social Workers, the Boy Scouts of America, the YMCA and the Hawai'i Business Jaycees.

Additionally, an important focus of *Sariling Gawa* has been to encourage and support higher educational achievement of Filipino students. Filipinos' educational attainment at the bachelor's level is lower than the population at large, 17.8% total population versus 12.6% Filipino population (U.S. Census Bureau, 2000). As stated earlier, youth leaders trained in *Sariling Gawa* have become professionals, contributing to the economic strength of the Filipino community as teachers, educators and lawyers. This is a major accomplishment given the fact that initially, Filipinos were brought to Hawai'i to work in the sugar cane and pineapple plantations and paid meager wages (Agbayani, 1996; Alegado, 1991; Cordova, 1983).

## *CONCLUSION*

This case study has illustrated that *Sariling Gawa* has ingredients of being a sustainable youth-run leadership development program. Filipino youth are the leaders of an organization whose mission is to work towards improving their own social, educational, health and overall well-being. *Sariling Gawa* is a community resource in Hawai'i that has developed, nurtured and sustained a substantial youth leadership. In a social environment where Filipino youth continue to feel discriminated against in society and feel that they have limited prospects in their schools or larger Hawaiian civil society to act as leaders, *Sariling Gawa* fills in the gaps by creating these opportunities.

Community based youth leadership development programs such as *Sariling Gawa* have a definite place within the Filipino and U.S. community, given recent census statistics. As stated earlier, Filipinos are a significant population among Asian Americans and the Filipino youth cohort has grown at a rate of 700% over the previous thirty years. Projections from the U.S. census data of the Filipino American population have indicated that this population's adolescents and young adults will predominate for at least the next two decades (Fawcett, Carino & Arnold, 1985; Ignacio, 1993). This young cohort faces the challenge of providing a stable and strong economic and social infrastructure for the rest of the Filipino American community. It is thus imperative at this stage of community growth and development that Filipino young people achieve overall physical, economic and social well-being.

Through *Sariling Gawa*, Filipino youth in Hawai'i have created a strong foundation for ongoing social change towards improving the living conditions for the whole community. However, in 2005-2006, as *Sariling Gawa* moves into the next quarter of a century of youth leadership development, the next steps will be to advocate for societal-level changes that would address deeper levels of institutional discrimination that leads to economic, social and educational barriers, as noted by Agbayani (1996) and Revilla (1996).

## REFERENCES

Agbayani, A.R. (1996). Education of Filipinos in Hawai'i. In Okamura, U.Y. & Labrador, R.N. (Eds.), *Pagdiriwang 1996: Legacy and vision of Hawai'i's Filipino Americans*. Honolulu, HI: University of Hawaii, Manoa.

Alegado, D.T. (1991). The Filipino community in Hawaii: Development and change. In Okamura, J.T., Agbayani, A.R. & Kerkvliet, M.T. (Eds.), *Social process in Hawaii: The Filipino American experience in Hawai'i. In commemoration of the 85th anniversary of Filipino immigration to Hawai'i. Volume 33*. Honolulu, HI: Department of Sociology, University of Hawai'i at Manoa.

Asuncion, L, Domingo, W., Macugay, M., Saludes-Galvez, A., & Los Banos, D. (1981). *Sariling Gawa (our own work): "Present and future challenges of Filipino young adults": A conference series*. Honolulu, HI: *Sariling Gawa*.

Berkman, L.F. & Syme, S.L. (1979). Social networks, host resistance, and mortality: A nine-year follow-up study of Alameda County residents. *American Journal of Epidemiology, 109*, 186-204.

Centers for Disease Control & Prevention. (2002). *2001 Hawaii youth risk behavior survey report-summary tables*. Honolulu, HI: Hawai'i State Dept. of Education.

Chesney-Lind, M., Marker, N., Rodriguez-Stern, I., Song, V., Reyes, H., Reyes, Y., Stern, J., Taira, J., & Yap, A. (1992). *Gangs and delinquency in Hawaii*. Honolulu, HI: Center of Youth Research. Social Science Research Institute. University of Hawai'i at Manoa.

Chesney-Lind M., Leisen, M.B., Allen, J., Browne, M., Rockhill, A., Marker, N., Liu, R., & Joe, K. (1995). *Crime, Delinquency and Gangs in Hawaii: Evaluation of Hawaii's Gang Response System Part 1.* Honolulu, HI: Center for Youth Research, University of Hawai'i at Manoa.

Cordova, F. (1983). *Filipinos: Forgotten Asian Americans.* Seattle, WA: Demonstration Project for Asian Americans.

DuBois, D.L., Felner, R.D., Felner, Brand, S., Adan, A.M., & Evans, E.G. (1992). A prospective study of life stress, social support and adaptation in early adolescence. *Child Development, 63,* 542-557.

Easterling, D., Gallagher, K., Drisko, J. & Johnson, T. (1998). *Promoting health by building community capacity: Evidence and implications for grantmakers.* Denver, CO: The Colorado Trust.

Erikson, E. (1968). *Identity: Youth and crisis.* New.York, NY: W. W. Norton & Company.

Fawcett, J.T., Carino, B.W., & Arnold, F. (1985). *Asian-Pacific Immigration to the ·United States. A conference report.* Honolulu, HI: East-West Population Institute, East-West Center.

Gao, G. & Perrone, P. (2004). *Crime in Hawai'i 2003: A review of uniform crime reports.* Honolulu, HI: Hawai'i State Attorney General, Research & Statistics Branch, Crime & Justice Assistance Division.

Gutierrez, L., Parsons, R., & Cox E. (Eds.). (1998). *Empowerment in social work practice: A sourcebook.* Pacific Grove, CA: Brooks/Cole Publishing Company.

Ignacio, A. (1993). Filipino Americans: A national, state and local profile. *Bigayan.* Filipinos for Affirmative Action. Oakland, CA.

Kuo, W.H. & Tsai, Y.M. (1986). Social networking, hardiness and immigrants' mental health. *Health and Social Behavior, 27,* 133-149.

Levitt, M.J. & Levitt, J.L. (1994). Social support and achievement in childhood and early adolescence: A multicultural study. *Journal of Applied Developmental Psychology, 15,* 207-222.

Luluquisen, E.M. (2001). *Sariling Gawa: Our own work. an evaluative case study of a youth-directed, community based program for Filipino youth.* Doctoral dissertation, University of California, Berkeley, School of Public Health. Dissertation Abstracts International. 63:03. Sept. 2002.

National Research Council. (2002). *Minority students in special and gifted education.* (M. S. Donovan & C. T. Cross, Eds.). Washington, DC: National Academy Press.

Parks, S. (1999). Reducing the effects of racism in schools. *Educational Leadership, 56(6),* 14-18.

Pearson, R.S. & Oliveira, C.M. (2002). *Ka Leo O Na Keiki: The 2002 Hawaii student alcohol, tobacco, & other drug use study: Adolescent prevention & treatment needs assessment. Filipino students.* Kapolei, HI: State of Hawai'i Department of Health, Alcohol & Drug Use Division.

Phinney, J. & Rosenthal, D. (1992). Ethnic identity in adolescence: Process, context, and outcome. In G. Adams, T. Gullotta, & R. Montemayor (Eds.), *Adolescent identity formation* (pp. 145-172). Newbury Park: Sage Publishers, Inc.

Revilla, L.A. (1996). Filipino Americans: Issues of identity in Hawai'i. In Okamura, J.Y. & Labrador, R.N. (Eds.), *Pagdiriwang 1996: Legacy and Vision of Hawaii's Filipino Americans.* Honolulu, HI: University of Hawai'i at Manoa.

Stake, R.E. (1995). *The art of case study research*. Thousand Oaks: Sage Publishers, Inc.

Stake, R.E. (1994). Case studies. In Denzin, N.K. & Lincoln, Y.S. (Eds.), *Handbook of qualitative research*. Thousand Oaks: Sage Publishers, Inc.

U.S. Census Bureau. (2000). *Census 2000 summary file 4 (SF 4)–sample data* [Data file]. Retrieved June 30, 2004, from U.S. Census Bureau Website: *http://fact finder.census.gov/home/saff/main.html?_lang=en*

Utsey, S. O., Ponterotto, J. G., Reynolds, A. L., & Cancelli, A. A. (2000). Racial discrimination, coping, life satisfaction, and self-esteem among African-Americans. *Journal of Counseling and Development, 78(1)*, 72-80.

Yin, R.K. (1994). *Case study research: Design and methods, Second Edition*. Thousand Oaks: Sage Publishers, Inc.

Yin, R.K. (1993). *Applications of case study*. Newbury Park: Sage Publishers, Inc.

# Youth as Engaged Citizens and Community Change Advocates Through the Lexington Youth Leadership Academy

Melanie D. Otis, PhD

**SUMMARY.** The Lexington Youth Leadership Academy is a leadership development and community change program which has helped high school-aged youth develop into effective leaders in a diverse society. The author describes a multifaceted approach emphasizing education and dialogue about diversity, training in problem solving and leadership skills, adult and peer mentoring, and community collaborations. The program employs an empowerment approach that begins with youth leadership development skills training, and culminates in youth-driven community change projects that focus on social injustice and educational reform. *[Article copies available for a fee from The Haworth Document Delivery Service: 1-800-HAWORTH. E-mail address: <docdelivery@haworthpress.com> Website: <http://www.HaworthPress.com> © 2006 by The Haworth Press, Inc. All rights reserved.]*

Melanie D. Otis is Assistant Professor, College of Social Work, 651 Patterson Office Tower, University of Kentucky, Lexington, KY 40506-0027 (E-mail: mdotis00@uky.edu).

[Haworth co-indexing entry note]: "Youth as Engaged Citizens and Community Change Advocates Through the Lexington Youth Leadership Academy." Otis, Melanie D. Co-published simultaneously in *Journal of Community Practice* (The Haworth Press, Inc.) Vol. 14, No. 1/2, 2006, pp. 71-88; and: *Youth Participation and Community Change* (ed: Barry N. Checkoway, and Lorraine M. Gutiérrez) The Haworth Press, Inc., 2006, pp. 71-88. Single or multiple copies of this article are available for a fee from The Haworth Document Delivery Service [1-800-HAWORTH, 9:00 a.m. - 5:00 p.m. (EST). E-mail address: docdelivery@haworthpress.com].

doi:10.1300/J125v14n01_05

**KEYWORDS.** Youth engagement, prejudice reduction, social capital, community-based services, youth leadership, community collaboration, social change, social justice

Contemporary American high school students are faced with many challenges not experienced by previous generations. They are educated in a climate that is often veiled in a threat of violence, in communities that are undergoing constant change and struggling with self-definition. Within this social context youth must learn to interact with people from a myriad of different racial and ethnic backgrounds, religious affiliations, socio-economic backgrounds, cultures, and sexual orientations. These challenges are set against the backdrop of the already difficult experience of adolescent development and its accompanying questions concerning one's own self-worth, personal identity, and purpose.

For community leaders and agencies who work with young people, the effects of this difficult climate can be seen, in part, in the rise of youth violence and bullying, and the growing number of adolescents who have become disengaged from school, family, and community. Amidst these images, youth tend to be viewed as uncaring citizens and problems to be handled, rather than potential contributors to social and civic life (Checkoway et al., 2003; Zeldin, 2002). Yet, research examining the issue of youth engagement from the perspective of young men and women, finds that many youth feel ignored and disrespected by adults around them. Others who may wish to become involved in community change efforts feel that they are left without the guidance or incentives necessary to move toward active participation in civic life (Benson, Leffert, Scales, & Blyth, 1998). These feelings are further magnified by youths' distrust of adult leaders and a growing belief that there is little they can do to influence change in their schools and communities (Zaff, Malanchuk, Michelsen, & Eccles, 2003). Additionally, among their peers, adolescents can feel excluded, shunned, or even fearful due to prejudicial attitudes related to race, ethnicity, gender, religion, sexual orientation, and/socioeconomic status (Fisher, Wallace, & Fenton, 2000; Pilkington & D'Augelli, 1995). Collectively, these factors often leave youth feeling powerless and disconnected from their communities.

Many argue that the solution to the problem of youth violence and disengagement from civil life lies in educating and mentoring young people to become youth leaders in efforts to achieve community change (Yates & Youniss, 1996; Youniss, McLellan, & Yates, 1997). The approach presumes that adolescents who have greater respect for diversity, better problem solving skills, and an understanding of non-violent ways to address issues that affect their lives, will want to work to change the climate of their schools and communities (Pate, 1988). Additionally, encouraging young people to become involved in civic life today will increase the likelihood that they will continue to be active, socially responsible citizens in adulthood (Jones & Hill, 2003; Zaff et al., 2003). Bourdieu (1986) argues that such involvement is critical to the development of social capital and the creation of strong democratic communities.

Programs that successfully facilitate youth participation in community change tend to bring together elements of youth development, engagement, and leadership enhancement, by focusing on youths' attitudes and values, providing experiential learning, and instilling a sense of communalism among participants (Bigler, 1999; Pate, 1988). Finn and Checkoway (1998) found that exemplary community-based youth programs hold in common: (a) a high level of youth involvement focused on issues affecting their lives, (b) a focus on individual, organizational, and community development and capacity building, (c) collaborative partnerships between a diverse community of youth and adults, and (d) active efforts to increase knowledge and understanding of diverse cultures. Ultimately, the ability of youth to engage in meaningful community change activities is enhanced by programs that link attendance to youths' developmental needs with identifying, supporting and facilitating access to engagement opportunities (Edwards, Johnson, & McGillicuddy, 2003). Camino and Zeldin (2002) found that such programs generate self-perpetuating enthusiasm for participation in community change, as youth come to feel more confident with their skills and are encouraged by the support they receive from collaborative community partners.

In this paper I will provide a case study of one such program–the Lexington Youth Leadership Academy (LYLA)–that was developed by the National Conference for Community and Justice-Bluegrass region staff. My own involvement with the LYLA program has come as a result of my work as a program evaluator and research consultant for the National Conference for Community and Justice-Bluegrass (NCCJ-Bluegrass) for the past five years. I will begin with a discussion of the philosophical and theoretical framework that guides the program, and describe the structure and core curriculum areas addressed in the youth leadership development program. After a brief summary of the empirical analysis of the impact of the program in areas relating to personal development, prejudice reduction, civic responsibility, problem solving, leadership skills, and peer relations, I will focus on two Community Change Agent projects conducted by senior LYLA ambassadors during their final months in the program. Implications of these findings for future youth program development will also be considered.

## *LEXINGTON YOUTH LEADERSHIP ACADEMY*

The Lexington Youth Leadership Academy (LYLA) is a community-based program created through the collaborative efforts of the National Conference for Community and Justice-Bluegrass region (NCCJ-Bluegrass), Partners for Youth (a program sponsored by the Mayor's office), and the YMCA of Central Kentucky. NCCJ-Bluegrass, a non-profit organization in Lexington-Fayette County, Kentucky (2003 population estimate: 266,798; U. S. Census Bureau, 2004), is the primary organization responsible for all phases of the program. The YMCA of Central Kentucky and Partners for Youth, along with a number of other community agencies, support the program by providing adult mentors, as well as opportunities for volunteerism and participation in decision-making as part of agency boards of directors and advisory boards. The project was funded, in part, by grants from the John S. and James L. Knight Foundation and United Way of the Bluegrass.

The National Conference for Community and Justice (NCCJ), the parent organization of NCCJ-Bluegrass, was founded in 1927 (originally known as the National Conference for Christians and Jews). NCCJ-Bluegrass is the regional office that serves Central and Eastern Kentucky. NCCJ's primary mission can be summarized by this quote from the organizations web site– "fighting bias, bigotry, and racism in America, while promoting respect and understanding among all people" (NCCJ, n.d.). In 1998, the national office for NCCJ made a decision to reorient their efforts to achieve organizational goals and transition all programming activities to concentrate on developing inclusive leaders with the capacity to effect social change in a diverse world. To that end, youth leadership development has taken a prominent place in the agency's work.

The foundation of the Lexington Youth Leadership Academy is built on this same philosophy. Designed specifically for high school-aged youth, the program provides a myriad of training and educational experiences aimed at helping participants become more effective, more inclusive leaders in their communities. Specifically, program components are designed to move from a focus on personal growth, skill building in areas of leadership and conflict resolution, and increased knowledge and understanding of diversity-related issues, to application of these new tools in addressing real issues in the community.

The philosophical underpinnings and mission of NCCJ are evident in all aspects of the LYLA program. For instance, LYLA participants are called Ambassadors to underscore the fact that they are acting on behalf of their peers and the community, as well as the program. It is a concept that conveys both expectations of action and a level of responsibility that extends beyond oneself. In addition to paying attention to the use of language and concepts that convey the philosophy of inclusion and civic responsibility, the program is designed to give participants increasing levels of input into decision-making, along with increasing levels of responsibility for the output that results. Adults (program personnel, mentors, community leaders) provide information, training, guidance, and feedback, but LYLA Ambassadors make the final decisions about community change projects they wish to pursue and how their goals may best be accomplished. To further assure that these decisions represent the interest of the collective, not just the will of the most verbal, meeting guidelines and LYLA staff set the stage for consensual decision-making. Thus, the process of community-building and the importance of responsible and committed participation that are hoped to be enacted in the community are modeled and experienced within the group. Finally, the program utilizes an empowerment framework which suggests that a youth who is supported and encouraged to evolve in terms of beliefs and attitudes about diversity, and who develops better problem solving skills and increased self-esteem, will be better able to take those tools and use them to be an effective, thoughtful agent of social change (Checkoway et al., 2003).

### Program Structure and Process

Since LYLA is a community-based program, participation takes place after school, weekends, and during summer months. Ambassadors are required to complete a minimum of 6 trainings per year. Trainings focus on one or more of the core program objectives–development of leadership skills, reduction of prejudice, increased self-concept, and civic responsibility. In addition, involvement in any activity is viewed as an avenue to increased self-awareness and a stronger sense of belonging to the group and the larger community. Trainings take a variety of forms from structured workshops, guest speakers, and field trips, to participation in other NCCJ youth programming (e.g., People-to-People, Anytown, U.S.A.), and vary in length from as little as 4 hours for some workshops, to as much as five days for participation in the summer diversity camp (Anytown, U.S.A.). Additionally, partnerships with community organizations, local government, schools, and involvement of adult mentors, provide ongoing support for LYLA Ambassadors, and create numerous opportunities for engagement and collaboration. Ultimately, the program components provide the necessary building blocks to allow Ambassadors to pursue a collective effort that has long range implications for their peers and the community as a whole.

One of the key criticisms of programs designed to increase youth engagement is that they often fail to address the developmental needs of youth involved. As previously noted, it has been argued that many programs may fail to develop sustained change in youth leaders by failing to link growth and skill development with opportunities for community involvement (Irby, Ferber, & Pittman, 2001). Thus, the LYLA program addresses the process of leadership development in youth. To that end, the LYLA program is structured around an educational model that views the ability to think critically and act purposefully as the result of a learning process. The model identifies six steps in the process: (1) knowledge and skills acquisition; (2) comprehension of information; (3) application to new situations; (4) analysis of information; (5) synthesis of information to think abstractly; and (6) evaluation–the ability to support decisions based on information and prioritize decision-making (Bloom, Englehart, Furst, Hill, & Krathwohl, 1956). Utilizing this framework, the LYLA program moves through three phases: *Phase One* focusing on personal development and capacity building, *Phase Two* focusing on applying new skills in peer mentoring and hypothetical settings, and *Phase Three* which involves utilizing knowledge and skills to create community change. Each of these areas will be addressed in greater detail.

### LYLA Participants

The philosophy and the goals of the program also guide the recruitment process. In order to provide both a model of inclusion and experiential opportunities to learn from others who may have dissimilar backgrounds, the overall composition of the LYLA group was diverse by design. Potential participants in the program were recruited through several means: (1) schools, (2) existing community programs, and (3) existing National Conference for Community and Justice

(NCCJ) programs. The multi-pronged approach to recruitment provided a diverse group of participants who varied in terms of sex, race, ethnicity, religious background, socio-economic background, sexual orientation, and personal experience. Thus, youth involved in the program came from all private and public area high schools, programs designed for high achievers and programs designed for youth experiencing school or behavior-related problems, as well as individuals who had participated in some past programming with NCCJ. Specifically, at the start of the first year of programming, the demographic composition of the group (N = 75) was primarily female (n = 55, 73.3%), fairly equally split between Caucasian Ambassadors (n = 35, 46.7%) and Ambassadors of Color (n = 40, 53.2%), with an average age of 15.8 years. Additionally, the majority of program participants were Protestant (n = 41, 61.3%) and identified as exclusively or predominantly heterosexual (86.3%).

### Phase One: Developing the Knowledge and Skills

Although the current paper focuses on the ambassadors' involvement in the community change and what they learned as a result of that involvement, past research on youth engagement indicates that the quality of that experience is partially dependent on the knowledge and skills they bring to the endeavor (Edwards, Johnson, & McGillicuddy, 2003). Thus, initial activities address knowledge and comprehension of discrimination, prejudice, and sources of stereotypes, while also encouraging introspection and personal growth. As youth begin to increase their capacity through increased knowledge and the development of new skills, the program also works to increase awareness of social issues and to foster a sense of social and civic responsibility (Mohamed & Wheeler, 2001).

### Phase Two: Learning to Apply What You Know and Gaining Confidence

In the second phase of the program, youth help to facilitate many of the program activities in which they previously took part. For instance, the Anytown U.S.A. program is a week-long diversity camp that addresses many of the same issues that are part of the LYLA curriculum, including racism, sexism, ethnocentrism, classism, and social responsibility. Ambassadors who had previously attended the program as delegates (camp participants) in Phase One of their LYLA experience could return to the camp the following summer to act as camp counselors (peer mentoring and education). Similarly, they might move into the role of facilitator for the day-long diversity workshop called People-to-People.

### Phase Three: Bringing It All Together: Community Change Agent Projects

A primary goal of the Lexington Youth Leadership Academy is to assist youth in becoming agents of positive change in their communities. To that end, each senior participates in a Community Change Agent project with a collective of other LYLA Ambassadors. Specifically, senior LYLA Ambassadors took part in one of two projects during the 2003-2004 year: the Race Dialogues and Diversity project or the Youth News Team project. Although LYLA staff provided support and resources for the projects, each project was youth-driven, with LYLA Ambassadors ultimately responsible for deciding on the focus of the project and identifying specific goals and objectives they hoped to achieve.

### Race Dialogues and Diversity Forums

In 2002, NCCJ-Bluegrass, in partnership with the Kentucky League of Cities and the NewCities Foundation, created the Leadership Initiative on Erasing Racism which brings community leaders together to develop strategies for eliminating racism throughout Kentucky. Participants represent a myriad of areas including, government, business, faith, school, education, and media. LYLA Ambassadors participated in this effort as members of the Youth Sector of the Leadership Initiative on Erasing Racism. Their Community Change Agent project, entitled *Race Dialogues*, involved a series of LYLA Ambassador-led town meetings focusing on understanding the pervasiveness and impact of racism in the Lexington-Fayette County community. Ten LYLA Ambassadors participated in the series of five race dialogue sessions, along with other youth recruited from Fayette County Public Schools.

LYLA Ambassadors also led two public forum discussions involving school administrators, teachers, social workers, law enforcement agents, and other youth leaders from Central and Eastern Kentucky. One forum focused on increasing diversity awareness among high school students, and used the curriculum from the National Conference for Community and Justice's one-day workshop–People-to-People.

People-to-People is a program facilitated by two trained co-leaders, who utilize videos, small group discussion (8 to 12 participants), and action planning exercises to expose participants to the impact of prejudice and discrimination. Participants are then encourage to take what they have learned back to their schools and communities to effect change through the development of human relations clubs, diversity dialogues, and community service (McAlister, Ama, Barroso, Peters, & Kelder, 2000). The second forum, a community-wide Town Hall meeting, brought adults and youths together to discuss issues of diversity and inclusion and identify strategies to facilitate social change.

*Youth News Team*

The Youth News Team consisted of a group of seven LYLA Ambassadors who chose to address the issue of the achievement gap among minority and majority students in the Lexington-Fayette County school system. The process began with a brainstorming session where Ambassadors identified issues that they believed affect youth and the community. As ideas began to be explored, Ambassadors were encouraged to consider how the issue fit with the things they had been learning about discrimination, diversity, problem solving, and social change. If Ambassadors found themselves struggling to identify concrete ideas, program staff assisted the process by suggesting various areas that directly impacted the lives of participants and their families. Ultimately they decided to focus on a school-related issue that had long range and far reaching implications in terms of educational policy and youth development–the achievement gap between minority and majority youth. As part of the process, Ambassadors considered the potential impact that their project might have on their peers, their schools, and the quality of life in their community.

The Youth News Team model used a youth-as-researchers approach (Horsch, Little, Smith, Goodyear, & Harris, 2002). Ambassadors acted as investigative reporters, conducting numerous interviews of students, faculty, school administrators, and community leaders. Additionally, they reviewed current research related to the achievement gap issue. Finally, as part of the information-gathering phase of the project, the news team surveyed 368 students in the local schools. Data from their findings were disseminated through a variety of media events including a press conference, and radio, television, and print media interviews. Their 42-page, final report–*The Achievement Flap: A Student Investiga-*

*tion of the Achievement Gap in Education* (LYLA Youth News Team, 2004)–was distributed to the media, local government, and community and school-based agencies. The document included background information from past research on the achievement gap, quantitative and qualitative findings from the student survey conducting by the YNT, transcripts of interviews with high school students, teachers, and five prominent community and/or education figures, including the Secretary of the Kentucky Education, Arts and Humanities Cabinet, the chair of the Fayette County School Board, the co-author of a recent book on the achievement gap, the executive director of an independent non-profit organization focused on improving education in the state, and the chairperson of a community board addressing issues of educational disparity. Based on their acknowledgement that the goal of their efforts was primarily to "initiate a dialogue that supports young people and adults to have more informed discussions about the achievement gap and other pressing education policy concerns," the team members also included eight recommendations for continuing the discussion of the achievement gap. In addition to their initial press conference to announce the completion of the study, the team broadcast a series on public radio. Local news media organizations publicly praised their efforts and endorsed the project.

### Impact of Lyla Program on Youth: How They Changed

Due to the comprehensive curriculum of the program, youth were asked to commit to a minimum of two-years participation, with many ambassadors completing a full three years of programming. A group of twenty-one ambassadors graduated from high school at the end of Year-One and completed their commitment to the program at that time. All LYLA Ambassadors were asked to complete a pretest, midpoint evaluation, and posttest assessment as part of their participation in the program. Additional qualitative data related to participation in the final Community Change Agent projects was gathered in focus groups. Together this information provides a picture of the impact of the program on multiple levels, with an expectation that growth in individual areas relating to civic engagement and social responsibility will ultimately culminate in action.

## Community Change Activities:
## Initial Qualitative Assessments

Initial assessments of the impact of participation in community change activities were conducted through debriefings which followed each media event or community action activity. These discussions were tape recorded and transcribed for narrative analysis. In a focus group conducted the week after the completion of the Youth News Media project, Ambassadors discussed their experiences and feelings about the project. They talked about their motivations for choosing to participate in the activity, their thoughts and reactions to the experience, what they learned about leadership, community involvement and diversity as a result of their participation, and how they planned to use the information gained as a result of the experience. Qualitative data from the focus group indicated that youth involved in the project experienced a notable shift in their commitment to community change as their involvement in the project increased. Several focus group members indicated that they started the project with the feeling that it was just a task to be completed and expressed concern that their peers might fail to do the work necessary to successfully complete such a large project. One young man cited past experiences where planned action had turned into inaction, and expressed concern that the same would occur with this project. Instead, he said he found himself committing more and more hours to the project as the level of interest and enthusiasm increased. Several youth credited the involvement of LYLA staff and other project participants as important contributors to the shift in their own commitments.

Members of the Youth News Team also discussed feelings associated with encountering prejudice and discriminatory thinking within the community. They were able to identify ways in which their participation in LYLA educational training made them more cognizant of these issues, and prepared them to address the problem more directly. The news teams' report clearly identifies examples of overt and covert prejudice that they believe contribute to the social injustices underscored by the achievement gap. For some members of the team, this became particularly evident when white Ambassadors' authenticity to address the issue of the achievement gap was questioned. One member of the group elaborated on this issue as he reflected on the press conference where they presented their findings and recommendations. A middle-aged, white male in attendance repeatedly questioned the background of the youth, suggesting that they were the product of white privilege, or the exception to the achievement gap issue if they were a person of color.

Three times, different YNT members attempted to address the critique primarily focusing on two separate arguments–(1) that his assessment of their lived experience was inaccurate, and/or (2) that the mandate to address an injustice should not be the sole responsibility of those who are affected, rather it is a social responsibility for any concerned citizen.

The event highlighted a number of important pieces of information. First, their efforts to respond to the criticism leveled against them highlighted their evolution as community change agents. They had learned some things. Although too nervous at the time of the news conference to fully appreciate the quality and composure of their response, YNT members later acknowledged that they had surprised even themselves with their ability to speak effectively and accurately on the issue, and with the poise with which they responded to the challenge. Youth News Team members also gained increasing confidence as they interacted with community leaders, political officials, public school officials, and the media in a number of different venues throughout the project. In focus group discussions, several youth expressed a sense that adults started these interactions with what one Ambassador referred to as a "let's humor the kids" attitude, but seemed to shift to a more respectful approach when they "realized we had something meaningful to say" (male Ambassador, age 17). Youth seemed empowered by the experiences, as they recognized that their hard work and systematic approach to the achievement gap project armed them with knowledge and insight that legitimized their presence in the discussion.

Many of the youth involved in the LYLA program have graduated high school and moved on to college and other activities. Program staff attempt to maintain contact with graduates of the LYLA program via phone calls, letters, and email. In these exchanges, former Ambassadors often acknowledge an awareness that their participation in the program has affected them–sometimes more than they realized at the time of their involvement. While reactions to participation vary, one young woman's comments are particularly compelling. Elissa Johnson (personal communication, March 17, 2005), now a sophomore at Fisk University, writes:

> The lessons I learned about being a change agent helped me to invite change into my life. It is so simple, yet so daring, the biggest strides I have taken against discrimination and intolerance have been to make people stand behind their words. There is an accomplishment in getting people to attend a diversity workshop, but they all usually have an interest in the topic. It is when you meet

people where they are, in their own environment and challenge their beliefs, and ask them to justify their convictions. Programming is the beginning of something much bigger, it is the lesson in how to teach and be taught by those who agree with you and those who do not.

The former LYLA Ambassador further demonstrates her belief in the importance of social and civic responsibility through her choices as a college student. Since arriving at Fisk University she has been involved in a variety of campus activities, including mentoring programs and the Student Government Senate.

## Impact of YNT Project on Community Leaders

Many of the efforts of the LYLA Ambassadors were well received. Prominent individuals in the community participated in lengthy interviews, and responded to questions with thoughtful in-depth answers. Both the level of time investment and the quality of the recorded responses suggested that they took the youth and their project seriously. Arnold Gaither, chairperson of One Community/One Voice, a coalition of groups focused on education and equity issues in the community, acknowledged the importance of the youth engagement during his interview for the YNT report, saying, "I think there are many young people who are out there just waiting to get involved. But I think that what young people want and need is a vision. . . . Sometimes older people need young people to give us their vision" (LYLA Youth News Team, 2004).

Feeling that the model program had proved successful, NCCJ-Bluegrass recruited a second group of Ambassadors in 2004. When members of the newly constituted Youth News Team approached the Fayette County School Board to request support for a survey exploring parents' roles in student achievement, the group received full support by the school superintendent and board. The multi-pronged project includes surveys and focus groups involving students and parents, interviews with school officials, and background research on the issue. Currently, the group is engaged in the formidable task of collecting data from all 9th through 12th graders attending the area's five public high schools–approximately 9,100 high school students in all. Although the project is still in the data collection phase, the Fayette County School Superintendent and Board of Education, as well as the non-profit educational reform agency, the Prichard Committee, have requested that the

Youth News Team meet with them for a formal presentation and discussion of their findings when the project is complete.

*Preliminary Changes in Approach to Community Change Agent Projects*

As previously noted, the current Youth News Team of LYLA Ambassadors is focusing on the issue of parental involvement in youths' academic success. An enhanced component of the LYLA program mirrors this interest. When the first group of participants went through the program, parents were often involved in various projects, assisting and supporting the work of the Ambassadors. For the present group of participants, parental involvement is more integral to the program model, as parents work alongside youth in a collaborative process.

## DISCUSSION

Youth have long been identified as the hope for the future, while simultaneously being marginalized within their communities–communities that may often contribute to the development and maintenance of juvenile delinquency, academic problems, and youth disengagement (Garbarino, 1995). Ironically, research suggests that engaged youth are less likely to participate in risk behaviors, more likely to be academically successful, and more likely to continue to be involved in civic life as adults. In other words, the engaged young person contributes to the social capital and development of his/her community. Over the past decade an increased interest in youth participation and community change has fueled efforts to develop program models that enhance youth development and support youth to become community leaders and engaged citizens. Many of these programs, like the Lexington Youth Leadership Academy, bring together tools to enhance youth development, youth leadership skills, and youth engagement efforts, in hopes of bridging the gap between youths' skills to create community change and their desire to do so. A preliminary assessment of the program suggests that the approach is largely successful.

Moving disengaged youth from the periphery of civic life to becoming engaged participants in social change requires the collaboration of community organizations, institutions, and citizens (Mohamed & Wheeler, 2001). To do so effectively, youth programming must begin by balancing the psychosocial developmental needs of the adolescent with attention to the importance of social context–an awareness that youth live in communities, not agency programs. The establishment of community partnerships that adhere to a philosophy of shared responsibility for the social welfare and development of youth help to provide an ecological environment in which personal growth may occur (Barton, Watkins, & Jarjoura, 1997). Within this supportive context youth can be challenged to examine their values and beliefs, and learn to be advocates for social change and social justice within their communities. The link between socio-cognitive development and community engagement is further fostered by adult and peer mentors modeling socially responsible behavior. These efforts will mean little, however, if adults do not value what youth bring to the discussion (Camino & Zeldin, 2002).

In a study examining patterns of community service involvement from high school to college, Jones and Hill (2003) found young people were more likely to continue their participation in community service when they moved from viewing it as service to viewing their activities as social action for change. Community Change Agent projects such as the Youth News Team and Race Dialogues are examples of ways high school-aged youth can engage in meaningful social action within their communities. The issues these projects addressed–prejudice, discrimination, and educational inequities–are issues that impact the lives of young people every day. As such, for many adolescents and young adults, participation in community change challenges young people to reflect on their values and beliefs, their sense of self, and their personal responsibility to their peers and community. Thus, external action is consistently coupled with internal developmental processes, and increases the likelihood of becoming an enduring influence on social and civic behavior.

## LIMITATIONS AND FUTURE DIRECTIONS

The real impact of the LYLA program–on both participants and the community–is yet to be revealed. Preliminary findings suggest that the program had a positive impact on the youth who participated, and was welcomed by adults in the community, schools, and local organizations. It is possible that the specific products of the efforts of LYLA Ambassadors (such as the report issued by the Youth News Team) may have less impact than the actual involvement of youth in peer mentoring and organizational decision-making as they carry out various tasks and roles as part of their involvement in the program. As members of the first cohort of LYLA Ambassadors, the young men and women involved in these initial projects were making bold statements about the role of youth in community change. They stepped forward, not as people who believed they had all the answers, but as people who believed they were integral to the process of knowledge development and community action around issues of diversity and education reform (Sherman, 2004). Adults in the community–educators and school officials, government leaders, agency personnel, and other engaged citizens–have generally viewed youth as part of the problem, not part of the solution. Further assessment of the program needs to explore the extent to which these images have been impacted by the actions of the LYLA Ambassadors.

The long-term impact of participation in the LYLA program is also unknown. Past research suggests that engagement in programs that provide meaningful experiences for participants often leads to continued engagement in civic life in adulthood. Continued involvement in civic life may partially depend on whether past participation was primarily motivated by external factors (i.e., peer and/or family involvement, required service) or internal factors (i.e., personal values, past experiences, belief in social responsibility) (Jones & Hill, 2003). As a community-based voluntary participation program, LYLA primarily focuses on nurturing and developing those internal factors that encourage lifelong committees to community engagement and social change. Longitudinal follow-up studies will need to be conducted to explore ways in which participation in the program has affected the lives of young people who became LYLA Ambassadors.

## REFERENCES

Barton, W. H., Watkins, M., & Jarjoura, R. (1997). Youths and communities: Toward comprehensive strategies for youth development. *Social Work*, *42*, 483-493.

Benson, P. L., Leffert, N., Scales, P. C., & Blyth, D. A. (1998). Beyond the "Village" rhetoric: Creating healthy communities for children and adolescents. *Applied Developmental Science*, *2*, 138-159.

Bigler, R. (1999). The use of multicultural curricula and materials to counter racism in children. *Journal of Social Issues*, *55*, 687-706.

Bloom, B., Englehart, M. Furst, E., Hill, W., & Krathwohl, D. (1956). *Taxonomy of educational objectives: The classification of educational goals. Handbook I: Cognitive domain*. New York, Toronto: Longmans, Green.

Bourdieu, P. (1986). The forms of capital. In J. G. Richardson (ed.), *Handbook on theory and research in education* (pp. 241-258). Westport, CT: Greenwood Press.

Camino, L., & Zeldin, S. (2002). Making the transition to community youth development: Emerging roles and competencies for youth-serving organizations and youth workers. In T. Burke, S. P. Curnan, J. Erickson, D. M. Hughes, N. Leon, R. Liem et al. (eds.), *Community youth development anthology.* Sudbury, MA: Institute for Just Communities, Brandeis University.

Checkoway, B., Richards-Schuster, K., Abdullah, S., Aragon, M., Facio, E., Figueroa, L. et al. (2003). Young people as competent citizens. *Community Development Journal, 38,* 298-309.

Edwards, D., Johnson, N. A., & McGillicuddy, K. (2003). *An emerging model for working with youth: Community organizing + youth development = youth organizing.* LISTEN, Inc. Retrieved March 8, 2005, from http://www.atthetable.org/handout. asp?ID=221

Finn, J., & Checkoway, B. (1998). Young people as competent community builders: A challenge to social work. *Social Work, 43,* 335-345.

Fisher, C. B., Wallace, S. A., & Fenton, R. E. (2000). Discrimination distress during adolescence. *Journal of Youth and Adolescence, 29,* 679-695.

Garbarino, J. (1995). *Raising children in a socially toxic environment.* San Francisco, CA: Jossey-Bass.

Horsch, K., Little, P. M. D., Smith, J. C., Goodyear, L., & Harris, E. (2002). *Youth involvement in evaluation and research.* Issues and Opportunities in Out-of-School Time Evaluation. Harvard Family Research Project. Retrieved March 7, 2005, from http://www.gse.harvard.edu/~hfrp/projects/afterschool/resources/issuebrief1.html

Irby, M., Ferber, T., & Pittman, K. (2001). *Youth Action: Youth contributing to communities, communities supporting youth.* Takoma Park, MD: International Youth Foundation.

Jones, S. R., & Hill, K. E. (2003). Understanding patterns of commitment: Student motivation for community service involvement. *Journal of Higher Education, 74,* 516-539.

LYLA Youth News Team. (2004). *The achievement flap: A student investigation of the achievement gap.* Lexington, KY: National Conference for Community and Justice-Bluegrass Region.

McAlister, A.L., Ama, E., Barroso, C., Peters, R.J., & Kelder, S. (2000). Promoting tolerance and moral engagement through peer modeling. *Cultural Diversity, 6,* 363-73.

Mohamed, I. A., & Wheeler, W. (2001). Broadening the bounds of youth development: Youth as engaged citizens. Retrieved March 15, 2004, from http://www.theinnovationcenter.org

National Conference for Community and Justice. (n.d.). Mission Statement. Retrieved July 6, 2004, from http://www.nccj.org

Pate, G. S. (1988). Research on reducing prejudice. *Social Education, 52,* 287-289.

Pilkington, N. W., & D'Augelli, A. R. (1995). Victimization of lesbian, gay, and bisexual youth in community settings. *Journal of Community Psychology, 23,* 34-57.

Sherman, R. F. (2004). The promise of youth is in the present. *National Civic Review, 93,* 50-55.

United States Census Bureau. (2004). Annual Estimates of Population by County, April 1, 2000 to July 1, 2003. Retrieved March 23, 2004, from www.census. gov/popest/counties/

Yates, M., & Youniss, J. (1996). A developmental perspective on community service in adolescence. *Social Development, 5*, 85-111.

Youniss, J., McLellan, J.A., & Yates, M. (1997). What we know about engendering civic identity. *American Behavioral Scientist, 40*, 620-631.

Zaff, J. F., Malanchuk, O., Michelsen, E., & Eccles, J. (2003). *Promoting positive citizenship: Priming youth for action.* Center for Information and Research on Civic Learning and Engagement, Circle Working Paper 05.

Zeldin, S. (2002). Sense of community and adult beliefs towards adolescent and youth social policy in urban neighborhoods and small cities. *Journal of Youth and Adolescence, 31*, 331-342.

# The Hampton Experience as a New Model for Youth Civic Engagement

## Cindy Carlson, MEd

**SUMMARY.** A commitment to engaging young people in civic life and public decision-making in Hampton, Virginia has inspired a model for youth civic engagement. The article presents two ingredients for successfully engaging youth: creation of a system of multiple engagement opportunities, and systematic efforts to address adult attitudes that fail to recognize young people as resources to their communities. The author analyzes the lessons learned from working within a system of youth civic engagement, and presents preliminary findings of the benefits of engaging young people in the civic life of a city. *[Article copies available for a fee from The Haworth Document Delivery Service: 1-800-HAWORTH. E-mail address: <docdelivery@haworthpress.com> Website: <http://www.Haworth Press.com> © 2006 by The Haworth Press, Inc. All rights reserved.]*

**KEYWORDS.** Youth engagement, youth as resources, youth participation, civic engagement, community building

### A NEW MODEL FOR YOUTH CIVIC ENGAGEMENT: THE HAMPTON EXPERIENCE

May 19, 2004. Members of one of Hampton, Virginia's largest and most influential commissions are gathered in the conference

Cindy Carlson is Director, Hampton Coalition for Youth (E-mail: ccarlson@ hampton.gov; Web: http://www.hampton.gov/for youth).

[Haworth co-indexing entry note]: "The Hampton Experience as a New Model for Youth Civic Engagement." Carlson, Cindy. Co-published simultaneously in *Journal of Community Practice* (The Haworth Press, Inc.) Vol. 14, No. 1/2, 2006, pp. 89-106; and: *Youth Participation and Community Change* (ed: Barry N. Checkoway, and Lorraine M. Gutiérrez) The Haworth Press, Inc., 2006, pp. 89-106. Single or multiple copies of this article are available for a fee from The Haworth Document Delivery Service [1-800-HAWORTH, 9:00 a.m. - 5:00 p.m. (EST). E-mail address: docdelivery@haworthpress.com].

room of a downtown public building. On the agenda this evening is a re-cap of the "highlights and lowlights" of the past year. The group runs through a series of accomplishments: successful advocacy for inclusion of a new facility in the Capital Improvement Plan; appropriation of over $35,000 in grant funds to community-based groups; a City Council Candidates' Forum so successful that it became a model for other sponsoring groups' forums. Then a realistic analysis of the negatives: a drop in attendance at public meetings; communication problems among sub-committees; lack of feedback on the group's input to the School Investment Panel. From all appearances, this could be a typical meeting on a typical night in the civic life of any city.

Now imagine that in the above scenario, the commissioners are clad in jeans and flip flops, munching on chips. Imagine their backpacks, jammed with homework, strewn about the floor, and parents in the parking lot waiting to drive them home. Yet, despite their young age, these commissioners are discovering a new voice and a new role in their community.

## AN EMERGING FIELD

There is a growing movement across the country that engages young people as active contributors to their communities. Terms such as "community youth development" (Hughes & Curnan, 2000), "youth organizing" (Funders Collaborative on Youth Organizing, 2000), "youth civic engagement" (Skelton, Boyte, Leonard, 2002), "youth infusion" (Lesko, 2001) and youth participation have gained considerable currency. Researchers and practitioners alike have documented and articulated the growing field and forged a new discussion on youth as participants in, and contributors to, community life and the democratic process. As a youth development strategy, the benefits of youth engagement to participants have been well-documented (Youniss, McLellan, & Yates, 1997; Pancer, 2001). Emerging research (Zeldin, 2000) now points to the impact of youth engagement on programs, systems and communities.

According to Sirianni and Friedland (2001), "American society needs to revitalize and modernize its civic infrastructure over the coming decades if it is to grapple with the increasingly complex problems of a world undergoing rapid transformation." They propose a civic renewal movement in which "we as citizens" are people who are "capable of engaging in complex public work and deliberation" acting as co-creators of policy rather than seeing themselves as victims of it.

We have learned from our experience in Hampton that this new view of "we as citizens" must undergo an even more profound re-definition to encompass those under the voting age. Since reinventing our civic infrastructure to include young people as essential contributors to complex public work, we have discovered that the true value of their engagement lies in its impact on the overall quality of life of the community. We have learned that we do not *want* them "at the table" because they are our future leaders (although prepared and trained leaders are a significant by-product of the experience). We *need* them at the table because they contribute a unique perspective today. They alone have the experience of living as young people in this time and place. And when provided with the necessary training and opportunities, their contribution results in better planning, better decisions, better programming, and better government.

In Hampton, where we use the term "youth engagement," young people have meaningful roles as service providers, advisors and co-creators of public policy, tapping both their innate interest in community life and their passion for improving it. Over the past decade our community's "table" has grown, first to accommodate, then welcome, more and more of its citizens. Young people, initially the most disenfranchised group, have emerged from their role of merely recipient of services to also become active participants in policy and planning. This journey has been a challenging one; a true shift of paradigm and a stretch of both young people's and adults' capacity to create and tolerate real change (Carlson, 2004).

## ONE COMMUNITY'S JOURNEY

Hampton's first community-wide planning process to determine strategic investments for youth took place in 1990. Faced with a declining economy and an increase in negative outcomes for its youngest citizens, City Council created a Coalition for Youth to develop recommendations that would make the city a better place for children and families. The first room was filled with "the usual cast of characters"–city leaders with decision-making authority over youth policy and programming. Years of experience and successful innovations had prepared us to respond to the challenge, yet also threatened to blind us to potential new solutions. Recognizing this, some members suggested that insight into the issues faced by our youth and families might be found outside the room. A comprehensive planning and outreach process ensued.

Five stakeholder groups were identified: parent; business; community/civic; youth worker and advocate; and youth themselves. One initial challenge was to create a group of diverse and representative young people who could provide much-needed insight into the opportunities and barriers perceived by teens. Although a review of the literature yielded few models to guide us, our intuition told us that youth in difficult life situations could serve as "experts" on those situations within a community planning process. Thus we combed the community for a representative sample of young people facing a range of barriers in their lives, who were surviving and even succeeding. For over a year, this youth group studied, debated, fought, listened, and struggled to articulate a vision for youth in their city. Most importantly, they taught a group of community leaders to listen and to hear the meaning behind their youthful words. In some cases issues topping the youth list did not surface in adult groups until adults recognized the wisdom of the young people's observations.

The stakeholder groups contacted over 5,000 of their peers to determine strategies that would ensure the health and success of local youth. The resulting Plan of Action (Hampton Coalition for Youth, 1993), adopted by City Council, provided the resources, policies, and commitments to sustain a long-term investment in youth, supporting them in their efforts to serve as resources to the community. It recommended a city-wide youth development approach which, through extensive capacity-building and service-learning components, would recruit and prepare young people for leadership, and train them, along with adults, to work in partnerships to address issues of local concern. The Plan included a policy statement, *A Community Commitment to Youth*, pledging that "All young people in Hampton are entitled to be seen, heard, and respected as citizens of the community. They deserve to be prepared, active participants in community service, government, public policy, or other decision making which affects their lives and their well-being." With this ringing endorsement, a youth civic engagement initiative was born.

The youth civic engagement system that emerged over the next 12 years–involving more than 15,000 of Hampton's young people in neighborhood, school, and community partnerships–can serve as a model for youth participation and community change. It is based on two critical elements shaped from our experience and desire to integrate young people into the fabric of civic life: (1) it is essential to construct an ever-expanding system of meaningful opportunities that can attract and engage the greatest number of youth in the broadest spectrum of participation; and (2) the fundamental work of a youth engagement initiative is not with the young people themselves, but with the long-held adult perspective that views youth as recipients of knowledge and services rather than resources to the ongoing challenge of building community.

## CREATION OF A MODEL OF YOUTH CIVIC ENGAGEMENT

We discovered our first premise of youth engagement quite by accident. The adoption of the 1993 Plan spurred a flurry of youth opportunities in Hampton's schools and neighborhoods. Alternatives, Inc., a local non-profit agency already recognized for their work in youth development and training, was selected to staff the initiative. Their staff recruited and trained hundreds of youth to be organizers, planners and change agents. Soon young people were painting aging houses, establishing tutoring and baby-sitting programs, looking in on elderly residents and joining civic associations. Some built successful partnerships with police officers and began to tackle neighborhood crime. The Superintendent of Schools convened a group of students to advise him on issues related to student life and school climate. The city's Director of Planning, witnessing the positive and immediate impact young people were having on planning processes throughout the city, decided to employ teenagers in his department. These Youth Planners contacted hundreds more of their peers in focus groups to gather input on the issues important to improving the city for its youth.

The further we delved into the work, the more we discovered about the fundamental qualities of young people's civic engagement. We knew that when an issue is important to them, young people will participate. But, just as with adults, teenagers' interest in civic affairs noticeably spanned a broad range from one-time volunteer opportunities to long-term commitments. For example, many youth were interested in issues related to transportation, especially bicycles. Within that group of interested youth, a large number welcomed opportunities to spend a Saturday morning teaching bicycle safety to children at a Bike Rodeo. Others would sign a petition or attend a public forum to speak out about a dangerous intersection. Some were thrilled to pore over street maps and create, alongside city planners, a proposal for a new bike route. And a few were inspired to research, write, and propose a new bicycle ordinance for the city. Over time our community's understanding of youth participation grew as a result of paying increased attention to the variety of ways young people respond to issues, and then challenging ourselves to explore with them new roles and opportunities.

Another discovery was the natural progression of many young people into increasing layers of complexity of civic commitment. In many cases, this appeared to be developmental; middle school-aged youth were attracted to the concrete, short-term experiences of community service while high school seniors were comfortable with the more abstract tasks of policy development. However, as we witnessed the increased participation of hundreds of youth, we noticed their corresponding development of capacity for tackling social issues. Despite their age or initial level of interest, many would gravitate over time to opportunities for greater impact and the increased challenges and responsibilities of engagement.

Then in 1999, while preparing for a visit from out-of-town guests interested in our fledgling initiative, a team of youth and adults created a graphic description of the roles young people were playing throughout the community. This graphic, however simple at first glance, has grown to illustrate Hampton's concept of youth civic engagement and incorporate our ever-increasing lessons learned about how practice becomes systemic.

### The Triangle Model

Within any civic engagement opportunity, people choose to participate at varying levels, depending on interest, availability, skill, or the ultimate goal of the activity in which the participant is engaged. For young people it is no different; yet, most adults limit their vision of teenagers' level of interest and their potential to help others or impact the community (Irby, Ferber, & Pittman, 2001). Thus, we propose a model of youth engagement with multiple pathways, represented by three layers of a triangle (see Figure 1). The three pathways, beginning with the base, describe an increase in the complexity of the role of the young person as an engaged citizen and a corresponding potential for impact on community change.

### Projects, Tasks, and Service

The myriad volunteer activities available to young people to be helpful and serve others constitute the first pathway of our triangle. Most communities have a host of these opportunities, scattered throughout

FIGURE 1. Hampton's Model of Youth Civic Engagement

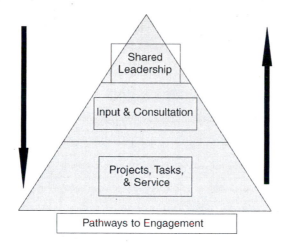

the youth-serving and civic institutions. They are short-term, often "hands on," activities requiring few specific skills and minimal training. The Projects Pathway can offer an almost unlimited variety of options for participation with specific issues that offer a positive experience to individuals. Young people participating in projects, tasks, and service can pass out campaign literature, collect canned goods for a food drive, conduct surveys, organize neighborhood clean-ups and recruit their peers to get involved. They are making a difference by giving of their time and talent or providing a needed service to the community.

### *Input and Consultation*

This pathway is an advisory function. Here young people enhance the decision-making and problem-solving of adults by adding a "youth voice" into processes usually dominated by an adult perspective. Although adults ultimately maintain the authority to decide, the unique perspective provided by young people impacts those decisions. Advisory opportunities can be short or long-term commitments, generally requiring skills in listening, presentation, and analysis of the issues in question, which may be broad or specific in nature. Where Project Pathway activities often impact an individual who is the recipient of a community service such as tutoring or volunteering in a nursing home, Input Pathway activities usually impact groups or organizations that benefit from the input provided. Youth-serving organizations, schools, and local government may provide opportunity for advisory-based engagement in the form of focus groups, advisory boards, "speakouts," and opportunities to assist in data analysis and program development.

### Shared Leadership

This pathway offers the greatest potential for impact on community change. Here youth work "shoulder to shoulder" with adults, sharing responsibility for activity and outcome. Many take on leadership roles far beyond those normally afforded others of their age, thus changing community norms of who is "at the table." This type of engagement carries a greater need for skill and commitment, and usually implies a focus on broader areas of impact–policy, strategic planning, systems change. Young people in the Shared Leadership Pathway may work within systems as board members or paid employees, or outside of systems as lobbyists or activists. Wherever they choose to focus their energies, they become part of deliberative processes focused on the decision-making that impacts the lives and well-being of youth and their communities.

Each pathway is an important element in an overall system of youth engagement. Whether the system encompasses an entire community, or is reflected within an organization or a grass roots initiative, the same principles of the triangle apply. The arrow on the left side of the diagram points to an increase in potential opportunities offered and the corresponding number of potential participants. The arrow on the right indicates the increased potential for community change and the corresponding need for higher levels of skill. While the number of individuals tends to decrease with opportunities further up the triangle, the potential for impact increases.

Communities and organizations wanting to increase the number of youth involved would be well served to include all three pathways of activity. Not only does this increase the possibility of attracting the greatest variety and number of youth, it increases the potential for impact on multiple issues of social concern. Just as in the bicycle example described earlier, within almost any topic of interest to youth, there can be a place for everyone and a variety of roles that contribute to community change. A sample of opportunities in Hampton's current youth civic engagement system is outlined in Figure 2.

An important lesson emerged from our Hampton initiative: view the triangle as a hierarchy of opportunity rather than a hierarchy of individ-

FIGURE 2. Hampton's Youth Civic Engagement Examples, 2004

| Projects, Tasks, and Service | Input and Consultation | Shared Leadership |
|---|---|---|
| Community service projects within a variety of school and community-based clubs and organizations<br>Curriculum-based service learning in school and after-school settings<br>Youth-to-youth mentoring<br>Youth Speakers Bureau<br>Neighborhood Youth Engagement Teams<br>Hearts to Hands–school/parent/community service projects<br>Youth-led volunteer projects<br>Youth website design and maintenance<br>Youth activism grants<br>Teen event planning<br>Red Cross youth prepared to assist in emergencies<br>KidsVoting Project | Superintendent's Student Advisory Group<br>Principal's Student Advisory Groups (all secondary schools)<br>Recreation Department Youth Advisory Groups (community centers, teen activities council)<br>Alternatives, Inc. Youth Advisory Board<br>Mayor's Committee on People with Disabilities (student advisors)<br>Community "speakouts"/youth public forums<br>Youth Task Force for School Investment Panel<br>Volunteer Center Youth Advisory Council<br>Neighborhood Youth Advisory Board<br>Developmental Assets Mobilization youth team | Youth-Community-Oriented Policing Effort (neighborhood & school-based partnerships)<br>Youth Planners (2 high school-age youth work in city planning department)<br>Hampton Youth Commission (all-youth policy level board)<br>Citizens' Unity Commission (youth voting members)<br>Neighborhood Commission (youth voting members)<br>Parks & Recreation Advisory Board (youth voting members)<br>Youth & adult training/consulting teams<br>Youth philanthropy<br>Teen center design and planning committee<br>Youth Component of 2010 Community Plan (youth responsible for community planning) |

uals with corresponding value placed on their level of engagement. Like adults, many young people want to participate only in the Project Pathway. Their desire for meaningful involvement may coincide with limited available time or different interests, yet it still must allow them roles as engaged and competent citizens. A strong foundation of these activities provides the scope of opportunities for youth to test their affinity toward civic involvement; the more opportunities, the more young people can find something of interest to them. This type of engagement is the very core of community-based volunteerism.

Once involved, opportunities open up for young people as they are exposed to new information, new skills, and new relationships. As they gain confidence, experience success, and taste the excitement of impacting change, their interest grows in the other pathways. If the scope of opportunities is crafted as a system, the likelihood for movement within the triangle increases. Often adults will notice youth volunteers who have passion for an issue and refer them to advisory opportunities. Young people who never considered board or commission work are introduced to public meetings by other youth. Youth in Shared Leadership roles are exposed to new volunteer service opportunities.

The result is a rich and diverse pool of youth leaders, passionate about their role in *their* community. Visitors to our community's youth engagement system marvel at the level of the work tackled by young people, but are even more amazed that they do not resemble a stereotype of youth leadership. Because a young person may have started in a neighborhood group and gained skills along the way, he or she may occupy a role that in other communities tends to attract only a few "superstars." We have learned to guard against assumptions that place young people in pre-determined citizenship roles, or practices that limit their access to any level of engagement in which they might be interested. As Irby, Ferber, and Pittman (2001) point out, young people must be exposed to multiple action pathways that provide "ongoing options for meaningful participation in organizations and activities that they believe will make a difference to someone."

## THE ROLE OF ADULTS IN YOUTH CIVIC ENGAGEMENT

Our work in youth engagement has been influenced significantly by the writing of William Lofquist, longtime proponent of community organizing on behalf of youth development. Lofquist (1989) presents a "Spectrum of Attitudes" describing a continuum of relationships, the attitudes of which affect the behaviors of one group of people toward another. The three relationships–Object, Recipient, Resource–correspond to a range of possible attitudes–particularly attitudes adults may hold toward young people. While all three attitudes can be appropriate depending on circumstances, the choice of one over another in a youth civic engagement initiative can result in young people feeling isolated and disenfranchised, or included and valued.

According to Lofquist, when adults view young people as Objects, the adult attitude suggests that they "know what's best for the young person" and have the right to determine the circumstances under which these youth function. For example, in public safety situations an Object attitude is necessary when an adult sets limits that will protect a child. Lofquist then contrasts the Recipient attitude in which an adult has something of value and believes that providing it to a young person will be good for him or her. Job training programs exemplify an appropriate use of the Recipient attitude when young people must learn a particular skill or portion of knowledge from the experienced adult. An adult with a Resource attitude believes young people bring something of value to a situation, such as a neighborhood planning effort, and that including them will enhance the adult's efforts. Many community situations are enhanced by approaching youth with a Resource attitude; however, problems arise when adults are mired in one of the other approaches and are unable to switch to new behaviors.

In the first two attitudes, the focus of the interaction is on the well-being of the young person—adults working on behalf of youth. In contrast, the objective of viewing another as a Resource is increased effectiveness, problem-solving and well-being of a group, community or targeted situation. Personal development and enhanced self-esteem of the young person, rather than the focus, tend to surface as byproducts of the experience of being treated as a Resource.

The Object, Recipient, Resource continuum, while deceptively simple, has been a rich source of learning for Hampton's proponents of youth engagement. While the language resonated with many of us, adult practice had yet to catch up with theory. Thus we discovered that organizations could become fluent in the language that described youth as recipients of their services, all the while youth continued to feel like objects when attending. Similarly, the more sophisticated the community became about the "youth as resources" concept, the more adults began promoting the value of youth involvement in decision-making and youth as partners. In many of these cases language, however important in describing intent, was not matched by behavior. The unfortunate beneficiaries of this problem were the youth who, seizing the opportunity for meaningful engagement, were disappointed when their input was not heeded or their participation not valued. In caution to other communities, we offer an expanded version of Lofquist's continuum (Figure 3).

Years of struggle with the implication of Lofquist's theory, observations of other communities and extensive dialogue with young people have led many of us in Hampton to conclude that adoption of a Resource attitude is a fundamental requisite for a successful youth civic engagement initiative. We have also learned that this requires a difficult shift in a community's culture that takes time, new skills, and a tremendous commitment by both adults and young people.

When youth engagement initiatives involve young people because "it will be good for them," the community risks missing the tremendous benefit of knowledge, skills, energy and insight of the youth. Unfortu-

FIGURE 3. Modified Spectrum of Attitudes Within Youth Civic Engagement

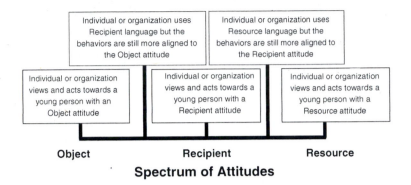

nately in many communities, children and adolescents are the necessary burden that adults need to manage until such time that they become valuable (adult). We have watched these communities fail in their attempts to create strategies that sustain youth engagement over time. In contrast, we have witnessed the incredible potential of youth as change agents in our community and in others, and noticed a corresponding value placed by those in power on accessing the contributions of youth.

Thus, a successful youth engagement initiative, with its focus primarily on improving outcomes for groups, organizations or communities rather than benefit to participating youth, will require as many adults as possible to adopt a Resource attitude and behaviors. Unfortunately, this is neither common, nor easy because many adults have learned over time to either dictate or abdicate responsibility when working with youth, and operate from long-held needs to fix, help, teach, and provide. A resume rich in youth work does not guarantee that an adult will function well in this new partnership role. Furthermore, youth are not accustomed to new roles as advisor or decision-maker, and many need a great deal of training and experience to shed their compliant or aggressive behaviors when interacting with adults.

Placing a single young person on a board or commission does little to advance the engagement of youth in a community, as it does not create access for large numbers of youth–especially marginalized youth–to decision-making, nor does it infiltrate the adult consciousness that would view them as valuable citizens. Some communities attempt to initiate youth engagement by creating board positions that often do little but create visibility for the attempt and, in the long run, reinforce stereotypes between youth and adults for whom the experience was a negative one. In fact, starting with shared leadership opportunities without the widespread exposure and intergenerational connections afforded by the triangle's other two pathways often leads to frustration and disinvestment by the community and the youth as well.

Our experience in Hampton has led us to believe that the level of skill, commitment, and passion exhibited by the youth commissioners in the opening scenario is only possible through this unique model of youth civic engagement and our adherence to the principles of recognizing them as resources to the ongoing process of building community.

## FINDINGS ON THE BENEFITS
## OF YOUTH CIVIC ENGAGEMENT IN HAMPTON

Good things happen when the role of young people is expanded within a democratic society. When youth become volunteers, advisors, and partners they become essential contributors to the civic infrastructure (Lewis-Charp, Cao Yu, Soukamneuth, & Lacoe, 2003). In Hampton we have recognized benefits from our youth engagement system in three primary areas: improvement in specific conditions; improved adult and local government decision-making; and increased social capital.

### Improved Conditions

When young people tackle a specific issue or social problem, their ideas and energy can contribute to improved outcomes related to that issue or problem. We have seen numerous examples of how this happens in our community. Early in our engagement initiative Hampton was experiencing a serious problem with juvenile crime in two low-income neighborhoods. Youth were perceived as problems by neighbors and police, and a widespread mistrust of law enforcement existed throughout the youth population. Our traditional approaches would have increased police presence, imposed curfews and surveillance, closed parks and playgrounds, and generally avoided contact with youth. Instead police, youth, and neighbors were brought together for team-building and training, and together the group created solutions. Youth and officers developed activities together, socialized, built relationships, and worked on crime prevention. At the end of the year, according to police data on reported crime, there was a 13% and 19% overall reduction in crime in the respective neighborhoods and an accompanying 44% and 54% drop in specific juvenile-related crime. Now youth serve on the civic associations and one of the neighborhoods was awarded the Governor's Excellence in Community Safety Award.

## Better Decisions

In countless situations over the past 12 years, youth input contributed to creative and successful solutions within local government and other community decision-making. When young people joined the neighborhood planning process in one of Hampton's older neighborhoods, adults were already divided on decisions regarding their most strategic investments–repairing the decaying infrastructure, investing in beautification to attract new business and home ownership, or supporting a proposal for a youth recreation center promoted by a vocal faction of residents. Teens in the neighborhood leadership group, with a similar passion to make their neighborhood a better place, were trained in communication and problem-solving skills and anxious to share ideas with their adult neighbors. Through the ensuing dialogue it became clear to adult residents and city staff that the young people did not support the recreation center proposal. Their vision of community involved lower cost options such as a neighborhood gathering place and intergenerational unity events. The resulting neighborhood plan built on the youth's vision and, according to city staff, potentially saved the city millions of dollars from an underutilized facility (Bayer & Potapchuk, 2003).

## Increased Social Capital

The neighborhood adults in the above example were introduced to a powerful new resource. City government staff learned a valuable lesson that investment in youth involvement brings a much-needed perspective to public deliberation. Similarly, schools, non-profits, congregations and businesses continue to benefit from the increased capacity of young people to contribute to the well-being of the city. This willing, yet previously untapped, group of citizens represents an increase in social capital. Our most recent administration of the Profiles of Student Life Attitudes and Behaviors Survey tells us that 40% of the teenage population engages in activities in one or more pathways of the triangle each year. From our annual tally of participants and opportunities, we conclude that an ever increasing number of neighborhoods, schools, youth services, and community organizations are benefiting from the energy and volunteer spirit of well-trained and committed youth. In addition to their leadership as current participants, we are also noticing a trend in their engagement once they become young adults. Many youth who participated as high schoolers in the late 1990s, according to staff observations, are returning to work in our youth engagement system or join new local civic initiatives. The movement appears to be "raising the bar" of expectations for youth as well as increasing the leadership pool of those who can meet those expectations. In a recent focus group of former participants, the now young adults spoke of a passion that was kindled in them as teenagers and the competencies they gained in their youth engagement experiences.

## CONCLUDING COMMENTS

Moving from a culture that views youth as objects, or recipients of what adults have to offer, to one that views them as valuable resources takes time and a tremendous commitment by both adults and young people. Adults must give away some of their long-held power and turf; youth must work hard to function effectively in the adult world. The results are worth the effort–we simply extend a caution that it won't be easy or quick. (Goll as cited in Carlson and Sykes, 2001)

For Hampton, the act and art of engaging young people in the civic life of the community has been both rewarding and challenging. Throughout our twelve years, we have also observed and supported other communities in their quest to create meaningful civic roles for their teen-age population, and have observed similar rewards and many more challenges.

We have learned that it is easy for communities to under-estimate the complexity of the process and the difficulties inherent in crafting a system of youth civic engagement. We have also learned that adults tend to under-estimate the power and potential of young people to address civic issues and social problems, often forgetting they are an important and willing stakeholder group. We have observed that when a community is not inclined to listen to and engage its adult citizens, it most likely will not value the engagement of its youth. When these challenges surfaced in Hampton it was important to use a thoughtful, reflective, and flexible approach to continuing the growth of the initiative and a tenacious attitude to keep the agenda in the forefront of the community. We also found that the best teachers of the above lessons are the young people themselves.

By far our greatest challenge is sustainability. Despite twelve years in operation, the initiative continues to struggle to overcome two major obstacles: succession and success. When City Council first adopted the recommendations that created youth engagement in 1993, the initiative's staff identified seventeen key community leaders whose support was critical for success. In the ensuing years, all seventeen of these individuals have changed, with some positions turning over many times. Each new mayor, superintendent of schools, or police chief brings his or her own interests and approaches, and the youth agenda must be re-visited and the support re-gained. Success can actually be a deterrent as well, as it is easy to give "lip service"–to assume that attention does not need to be paid to development or that funding is easy to obtain. Even more potentially damaging is the attitude that "we don't need to work on that anymore" and thus turn our attention to other issues. Again, the intentional and stubborn approach has served us well to educate community leaders to the necessity of an ongoing investment in each new generation of Hampton's youngest citizens.

Despite the challenges, engaging a new group of citizens in community building has for us been its own reward. This exciting and vibrant system of engagement opportunities for youth has become a fixture in Hampton's civic landscape. In post testing and exit interviews, participants in youth civic engagement report gaining the skills of public deliberation, presentation, and activism, and a passion for affecting community change. In conversations when they return, these young adults also express disappointment when their college environment or new community does not afford them the same opportunities. They report that their choice of a community to live in will definitely include a vibrant civic culture. Indeed, they may not tolerate a community that acts otherwise. Because of this, our community and others that have embraced this approach believe that we are creating a new norm for the next generation of a responsive, accessible government and a foundation for future civic engagement.

Based on our own experience in Hampton, and the successes and feedback from other communities with whom we have shared our ideas, the triangle model of youth civic engagement appears to hold strong implications for future practice. In addition, both the challenges and rewards of Hampton's experience in youth civic engagement mentioned above raise issues that warrant further study.

From our experience, we do know that it is possible to sustain and even grow a youth civic engagement initiative. While we have some observations regarding the community climate that has helped it to flourish, the study of similar attempts in less than promising climates would help to pinpoint the fundamental conditions that can support, or are necessary for, a thriving youth engagement initiative.

And while our experience tells us that engaging today's youth yields future benefits for them and for our community, we believe more long-term study on the benefits is warranted. Do the skills and behaviors of civic engagement carry over from youth to adulthood? Will active and engaged youth become active and engaged adults? Will their experience of an abundance of civic opportunities determine an expectation of a similar climate in their adult lives? And does investment in the civic engagement of young people result in the best and brightest of those youth returning to the community to re-connect with a place where they were valued as youth?

## REFERENCES

Bayer, M. & Potapchuk, W. (2003). *Learning from neighborhoods: The story of the Hampton Neighborhood Initiative.* Hampton, VA: Hampton Neighborhood Office.

Carlson, C. (2004). A rightful place: Expanding the role of young people in a democratic society. *The Good Society, 13,* 39-43.

Carlson, C. & Sykes, E. (2001). *Shaping the future: Working together, changing communities.* Hampton, VA: Hampton Youth Commission.

Funders Collaborative on Youth Organizing (2000). *An emerging model for working with youth.* (Occasional Papers Series, 1). New York: LISTEN.

Hampton Coalition for Youth (1992). *2 commit 2 the future 4 youth: A plan of action.* Hampton, VA: Coalition for Youth.

Hughes, D. & Curnan, S. (2000). Community youth development: A framework for action. *CYD Journal, I,* 7-11.

Irby, M., Ferber, T., & Pittman, K. (2001). *Youth action: Youth contributing to communities, communities supporting youth.* (Community and Youth Development Series, 6). Takoma Park, MD: Forum for Youth Investment, International Youth Foundation.

Lesko, W. S. (2001). *Youth infusion: Intergenerational advocacy toolkit.* Kensington, MD: Activism 2000 Project.

Lewis-Charp, H., Cao Yu, H., Soukamneuth, S., & Lacoe, J. (2003). *Extending the reach of youth development through civic activism: Outcomes of the youth leadership for development initiative.* San Francisco: Social Policy Research Associates.

Lofquist, W. (1989). *The technology of prevention workbook.* Tucson, AZ: AYD Publications.

Pancer, M. (2001, May). *Does research tell the whole story? Initial summary of the CEYE literature review.* Retrieved December 28, 2003, from *http://www.engage mentcentre.ca*

Sirianni, C. & Friedland, L. (2001). *Civic innovation in America: Community empowerment, public policy, and the movement for civic renewal.* Berkeley: University of California Press.

Skelton, N., Boyte, H.C., & Leonard, L.S. (2002). *Youth civic engagement: Reflections on an emerging public idea.* Minneapolis, MN: Center for Democracy and Citizenship.

Youniss, J., McLellan, J.A., & Yates, M. (1997, March/April). What we know about engendering civic identity. *The American Behavioral Scientist, 40*(5), 620-631.

Zeldin, S., McDaniel, A.K., Topitzes, D., & Calvert, M. (2000). *Youth in decision making: A study on the impacts of youth on adults and organizations.* Chevy Chase, MD: Innovation Center for Community and Youth Development.

# YOUTH PARTICIPATION IN EVALUATION AND RESEARCH

## Urban Youth Building Community: Social Change and Participatory Research in Schools, Homes, and Community-Based Organizations

Kysa Nygreen, PhD
Soo Ah Kwon, PhD
Patricia Sánchez, PhD

Kysa Nygreen is a President's Postdoctoral Fellow, University of California, Santa Cruz. Soo Ah Kwon is Assistant Professor of Asian American Studies and Human and Community Development, University of Illinois, Urbana-Champaign. Patricia Sánchez is Assistant Professor, College of Education and Human Development, University of Texas at San Antonio.

The authors would first and foremost like to thank all the youth in the East Bay who are working hard in their communities and bringing their knowledge, experiences, and cultural resources to the table. In addition, the authors are indebted to the Center for Participatory Research and Popular Education (CPEPR) at the Graduate School of Education, University of California Berkeley, which nurtured both a physical and intellectual space for this type of work.

[Haworth co-indexing entry note]: "Urban Youth Building Community: Social Change and Participatory Research in Schools, Homes, and Community-Based Organizations." Nygreen, Kysa. Soo Ah Kwon, and Patricia Sánchez. Co-published simultaneously in *Journal of Community Practice* (The Haworth Press, Inc.) Vol. 14, No. 1/2, 2006, pp. 107-123; and: *Youth Participation and Community Change* (ed: Barry N. Checkoway, and Lorraine M. Gutiérrez) The Haworth Press, Inc., 2006, pp. 107-123. Single or multiple copies of this article are available for a fee from The Haworth Document Delivery Service [1-800-HAWORTH. 9:00 a.m. - 5:00 p.m. (EST). E-mail address: docdelivery@haworthpress.com].

**SUMMARY.** "Urban" youth–a euphemism for underserved, poor, marginalized, ethnic minority youth–can be active participants in community change. Countering the predominant image of these youth as disengaged or troubled, this article describes three projects that engage urban youth in community change through participatory research. The authors share their experiences as adult allies on these projects and examine four lessons learned, addressing: (1) the importance of positionality; (2) the role of adult allies in youth-led projects; (3) the creation of safe spaces; and (4) the building of trust and relationships. They conclude that urban youth can become a vital resource for community transformation. *[Article copies available for a fee from The Haworth Document Delivery Service: 1-800-HAWORTH. E-mail address: <docdelivery@haworthpress.com> Website: <http://www.HaworthPress.com> © 2006 by The Haworth Press, Inc. All rights reserved.]*


**KEYWORDS.** Urban youth, participatory research, social/community change, youth leadership, race/class/gender/culture, adult allies


## *INTRODUCTION*

Increasingly scholars and policy makers are paying attention to the role of meaningful youth participation (O'Donoghue et al., 2002; McLaughlin et al., 1994), youth civic engagement (Youniss et al., 1997, 2002), and marginalized youth of color organizing for social justice (Ginwright & James, 2002; Ginwright & Cammarota, 2002). Our recent experiences as adult allies in efforts to engage youth in social change have helped confirm our long-held beliefs that "urban" youth–a euphemism for underserved, poor, marginalized, ethnic minority youth–can be important actors in shaping their schools and communities.[1] Despite a dominant discourse that frames urban youth as disengaged or troubled, our experiences suggest that these youth, if given the opportunity, can become competent citizens (Checkoway et al., 2003), active participants, and powerful agents of social change.

As former elementary and high school teachers, we hold a special stake not only in the realization of such youth-driven work, but also in the maintenance of a dialogue on this topic. Given the persistent failure of public institutions like schools to serve "inner-city" youth (Anyon, 1997; Aronowitz & Giroux, 1985; Fine, 1991; Noguera, 1996, 2003; Oakes, 1985; Payne, 1984), the promise of a better future for these youths' long-neglected and underrepresented communities needs to be re-directed toward the valuable human resources already present in such neighborhoods. The experiences and knowledge of African American, Asian and Pacific Islander, Chicana, Latino, white, immigrant, transnational, and minority youth can be a vital source in the transformation of their schools, homes, and the community-based organizations (CBOs) that work with them.

In this article, we investigate the role of participatory research as a model of engaging *with* youth for social change. We share the work we have carried out with three different groups of youth in northern California: PARTY–a multi-ethnic school-based group of students transforming curriculum at an alternative high school; TNL–a small group of Latinas conducting research in both their U.S. and Mexican "homes" on children's transnational experiences; and AYPAL–a pan-ethnic Asian and Pacific Islander CBO focused on youth organizing and social justice. We offer an illustration of these projects and some of their results, as well as a close look at the lessons learned through our participation as adult allies. Additionally, we examine our roles as university-based researchers *and* active participants in youth-led efforts for community change through the model of participatory research with youth.

## PARTICIPATORY RESEARCH AND YOUTH

> The purpose of participatory research is not merely to describe and interpret social reality, but to radically change it. (Maguire, 1987, p. 28)

We define participatory research as an alternative paradigm of knowledge production in which groups who are adversely affected by a social problem undertake collective study to understand and address it (Hall, 1992, 1993; Maguire, 1987, 1993; Park, 1999; Tandon, 1981; Vio Grossi, 1981). Participatory research is not just a "method" involving participation by research subjects: it "presents people as researchers in pursuit of answers to questions of daily struggle and survival; breaks down the distinction between researcher and researched . . . and returns to the people the legitimacy of the knowledge they are capable of producing" (Hall, 1992, p. 16).

Participatory research is usually carried out by people from marginalized communities such as the poor, immigrants, women, or people of color. It is based on the assumption that people are capable of understanding the social forces that shape the conditions of their lives. Research questions speak to the needs of the group because they emerge from their shared experiences. University-based researchers may participate as allies and contributors, but community-based members retain control over each phase of the research process, from developing research questions and methods, to interpreting and using the results as the basis for collective action.

Although we often do not think about age as an axis of oppression like race, gender or class, youth in fact represent a marginalized group in society (Laz, 1998; Males, 1999; Minkler & Robertson, 1991). Despite youth's marginalized status, the most widely-circulated texts on participatory research tend to focus on projects involving adults (e.g., Ansley & Gaventa, 1997; Fals-Borda & Rahman, 1991; Hall, 1992; Maguire, 1987; Park, Brydon-Miller, Hall, & Jackson, 1993). Thus, the distinct opportunities and challenges of doing participatory research with youth have not been sufficiently explored in the literature. This article seeks to amplify the literature on participatory research by focusing on the role of urban youth in these efforts. Our experiences confirm that youth-led participatory research can be a powerful way to engage urban youth as active participants in school and community change.

## THREE YOUTH PROJECTS

The youth-driven projects we have worked with have evolved and taken root in different social settings–a high school, homes, and CBOs. Yet the three projects are similar in two important ways: first, all three were conceived via an established relationship between adult allies and youth. In other words, much dialogue and community-building took place organically in the spaces we adult allies shared with the youth prior to initiating the research. Secondly, in all three projects, urban youth and their worldviews and concerns were at the center of the research and learning experience–unlike much of the youth's own public schooling experiences. Below we describe in more detail each project, pointing toward the powerful learning and social-change experiences created in these out-of-school settings.

### Participatory Action Research Team for Youth (PARTY)

The Participatory Action Research Team for Youth (PARTY) involves five recent graduates and current students from Jackson High

School[2] (ages 16-19), and myself (Nygreen),[3] a former Jackson teacher and university-based researcher (age 27).[4] Our shared community is a public alternative high school serving predominantly low-income youth of color who have been labeled "at-risk." Together we embarked on a participatory research project aimed at making change within the school. Our team represents diverse ethnic backgrounds including African American, Filipino, Latino, and white.

In the first year, PARTY met weekly to conduct collaborative research on social issues affecting the school community. In these meetings we engaged in group reflection and dialogue about social and political issues, learned new facts and information, shared personal experiences, and built relationships across age, gender, race, and class. We discussed how social issues and news events affected our lives and the lives of Jackson students. In order to learn more about how social issues affected the lives and education of Jackson students, we conducted a school-wide survey and carried out audio-taped interviews with school staff, teachers, and students.

The next year we applied our findings by developing and teaching a high school course at Jackson High. The purpose of our course was to inspire Jackson students to think critically about social justice issues and engage in action for social change, as one PARTY member explained, "I want to see people who have a positive spin on society and get out there and become *part* of society . . . contribute to what's going on in your country, . . . contribute to things being better." Our course was approved by the principal and social studies teacher, and we gained permission to teach a weekly, 80-minute lesson in the U.S. government class. PARTY members developed lesson plans and taught the class, employing dialogue-based pedagogy to address topics like police brutality, prisons, and environmental racism.

For the PARTY participants, teaching the weekly government class was a concrete action for social justice in our school community. In designing and teaching a high school class, PARTY members took on traditionally adult roles, gaining confidence and leadership skills, as one participant reflected, "I gained a lot of strength being in this group. . . . I realize that I can really be confident. . . . I've gained a lot more power in myself. And I can articulate a lot better."

### Transnational Latinas (TNL)

Transnational Latinas (TNL) has been working together for over three years. We are four Latinas–three youth (ages 13-16) and a graduate student (age 29) whose parents emigrated from small rural communities in México.[5] Utilizing participatory research, we have attempted to document and understand the lives of transnational immigrant children and families, ultimately sharing this information through a co-authored children's book.

I (Sánchez) first met two of the youth through work at a community-based family literacy program; the third youth I met through a yearly pen-pal letter program in a local school district. Upon learning that all four of us were traveling to México to visit family, we came together as a group to share our pictures and experiences on these yearly trips. For the first year of our project, we simply got to know each other more, to understand our families' ties to México, and explore the meaning this had in our lives as transnational second-generation female immigrants. We had often shared how our trips to México, language, and close-knit immigrant culture were rendered invisible in school. This led to our decision to write a children's book on what it was like growing up in two homes spread across an international border.

The youth and I conducted research on this type of life through: (1) dialogue, (2) interviews and field notes with transnational families in both the U.S. and México, and (3) a collection of documents, such as home videos, pictures, writings, and other items exchanged in transnational families. Throughout this process, our families in both California and parts of México were excellent supporters and resources. We took their knowledge as members of transnational communities and created a meta-narrative, as seen through a child's eyes, of what life is like in these places.

Finally, we spent the last twelve months of our project writing and illustrating our book. We printed the first 80 copies with money we received from a small grant at a local copy store and distributed these to our families, at teacher conferences, local libraries, and day care centers. Most recently, the same CBO–where two of the youth still work–connected us to a children's book publisher that is now working with all four of us on national distribution.

### Asian and Pacific Islander Youth Promoting Advocacy and Leadership (AYPAL)

The Asian and Pacific Islander Youth Promoting Advocacy and Leadership (AYPAL) is a pan-ethnic community-based youth organizing collaborative made up of six Asian and Pacific Islander (API) youth groups including Cambodian, Chinese, Filipino, Korean, Laotian,

Mien, Samoan, Tongan, and Vietnamese youth, ages 14-18. As an organization, AYPAL works toward accomplishing three overarching goals with their youth: building youth-led community groups, promoting youth civic participation and community leadership, and promoting self and cross-cultural understandings.

Unlike PARTY and TNL, AYPAL was not initiated as a research project. Rather, I (Kwon) became involved in an existing CBO's effort to engage youth in civic participation. I was immediately drawn to the politically active group and became a volunteer youth community organizer. Over time, I built authentic relationships with the staff and youth of AYPAL and became integrated as a member of the organization. I shared in the analyses, actions, and reflections organized by AYPAL and my role as a researcher has always been secondary.

Although AYPAL does not overtly identify as employing the principles of participatory research, they understand that knowledge production and solutions come from those who are adversely affected by social problems. Each year, AYPAL youth are engaged in a youth-led community organizing campaign that addresses a problem in their community that stems from their personal experiences. Campaigns include organizing for an ethnic studies curriculum to be taught in high schools; creating district-wide policy changes to address school police harassment, to unlock bathrooms during passing periods, and to require teachers to hand out written grading policies. AYPAL also convinced local city council members to increase programming and staff at neighborhood recreation centers and worked with a local congresswoman to sponsor a bill into congress that would end deportations of legal immigrants.

## LESSONS LEARNED

In this section we discuss four of the major lessons we learned as adult allies with PARTY, TNL, and AYPAL, which we believe best represent our shared experiences, and speak most succinctly to the power of these youth-led grassroots efforts.

### Recognizing Race, Class, Gender, and Culture

In much of the literature on youth and community participation, the role of race, class, gender, and culture is often glossed. Though some authors have referred to it in describing the work of organizations that see youth as "competent citizens" or "community builders" (Checkoway et al., 2003; Finn & Checkoway, 1998), we propose that more youth practitioners and researchers interrogate the issue of positionality–by which we mean the relative power, privilege, and position of all group members. Indeed, we have found that those who work with urban youth–or those who write about others who do–need to incorporate a more extensive discussion on how these social constructs play a critical and material role in working with communities of color. This applies to the role of adult allies as well as the overall youth-led projects.

In two of our projects, TNL and AYPAL, youth and adult allies shared similarities of race, immigration status, and social class. These common experiences facilitated initial entry into many of the immigrant youth's communities as well as their recruitment into the projects. For example, Kwon believes that her acceptance into AYPAL was easily facilitated by her position as a 1.5-generation Korean American. Additionally, the shared experiences and identities of the youth and adult allies helped reduce struggles of power and conflict within the groups.

These common experiences were also central factors in the way that TNL and AYPAL were organized and the type of work embarked upon. For example, the main goal of TNL–researching and writing about the way children experience "home" and transnationalism–was very much a central aspect of all TNL members' lives. Sánchez recognized the role of culture, language, and family in her work with TNL and immediately sought support of the project by the young women's families through face-to-face interaction. Maintaining relationships with youth's families in their home language enhanced the project. The cultural value of family, as experienced by Mexican immigrants, was also a remarkable resource in traveling to México and staying with relatives of both the youth and adult ally during the initial phase of data collection. AYPAL also recognizes the importance of young people's racial identity as second-generation Asian and Pacific Islander youth. Through workshops and cultural arts projects, youth link their racial and pan-ethnic API identities to a powerful political identity. This emphasis on youth's cultural and political history is often neglected in schools.

Yet in many youth projects, such as PARTY, the adult allies do not share the youth's racial, class, or gender backgrounds. Because PARTY participants initially knew Nygreen as their teacher, they often viewed her as an authority figure rather than an ally, partner, or colleague. Contributing to the perception of Nygreen as *teacher* is the fact that she, like most of the teachers at Jackson High, is white while the students at Jackson High are predominantly African American (approximately 75%). It therefore became important to construct a shared sense of community within PARTY and to address relations of power and privilege within the group.

The lesson learned for adult allies in youth-led projects is the importance of positionality as well as the adult's institutional relationship with youth. Adult allies must be conscious of the ways that race, class, gender, and culture can shape their relationship with youth. We must take into account both our formal, institutionalized relationship with youth, as well as the perceptions that youth have of the adult on the basis of this relationship.

### Strengthening Adults as Allies

Leading but not leading, is this possible? The challenge of leading without controlling is central in participatory research (Maguire, 1987, 1993). Ideally, participatory research projects employ democratic decision-making processes in which all members of the group share equal power (Gaventa, 1993; Hall, 1992). In reality, however, intra-group power inequalities and conflicts often emerge, and these frequently reflect larger societal relations of power and privilege (Maguire, 1993; LeCompte, 1995). In our experience, we have found that power inequalities between youth and adult allies are often masked through discourses such as "youth-led" and "youth-initiated" when in practice, these projects are heavily directed by adult participation. These struggles are especially pertinent because wider societal power relations between adults and youth or teachers and students are well established (Laz, 1998; Males, 1999; Minkler & Robertson, 1991). We address some of these issues of power in our roles as adult allies.

In PARTY, an important contradiction became evident once the youth began teaching the government class at Jackson High: here was a *youth-led* project in an *adult-controlled* institutional context, a public high school, where the parameters of possible action are defined by adults. This contradiction came to the fore when PARTY members, while teaching their class, brought students outside to play basketball as part of their relationship-building pedagogy. After class, the PARTY members were reprimanded for failing to get permission from the teacher for this activity. Thus, although the weekly government class was "youth-led," the PARTY youth were empowered only within the limitations of pre-existing (adult-defined) school rules, policies and procedures. These were in essence a set of "non-negotiables" that youth were bound to obey but could not influence.

For TNL, the opposite was true; the group was able to work on its own timeline with little or no institutional constraints. However, struggles between youth leadership and adult control still arose. As a former teacher, Sánchez struggled to maintain a balance of encouragement and guidance without domination. She found that just keeping silent more often during meetings granted others more time to think, participate, and express themselves as well as gain further ownership of the project. In addition, discussions of non-negotiables often came up in the course of traveling to México or to present at various out-of-town conferences. At other times, Sánchez offered her advice on some of the ways children's literature was used in the classroom by bilingual teachers. It was helpful to recognize that some adult knowledge *is* important in working with youth, and it would be disingenuous to not bring that forward.

AYPAL's adult leaders hold this belief as well. They understand that youth need to be guided by the expertise and knowledge that comes from their experiences as adult community organizers. One adult staff's comment shows how to find the balance between adult direction and youth ownership:

> If you let youth organize whatever they want to organize, they might organize a picnic or a dance. (Laughs) . . . It is hard finding the right balance, right? Because ultimately you do want the youth to feel it and they should make all the important decisions. But then you also want to recognize that . . . I *do* know more about organizing than they do. And there has to be some process where, you know, my wisdom and the wisdom of the other staff can be passed along to the youth and then the youth can make decisions.

Youth also see the role of adult coordinators in AYPAL as mentors, providing guidance for youth-initiated and youth-led community organizing projects. One youth explained:

> Like in AYPAL, you have the coordinator that teaches you. But the site coordinator is not really like your teacher, but they're just there to support you. Like they have us doing our own agenda, hosting the meetings with different youth, it's youth ownership. Like in high school, they [the teachers] boss you around and tell you what to do. . . .

Through our work with PARTY, TNL and AYPAL, we gleaned important lessons about the role of adult allies in youth-led projects. First, we found that non-negotiables are almost always present in work with youth, even if they are unstated. We propose that adult allies be upfront with youth about any non-negotiables or adult-led activities from the outset of the project and to let youth come up with their own set of non-negotiables as well. Secondly, we found that adult allies often have important knowledge to share with youth and should work to achieve a balance that ensures both youth leadership and adult contribution. Moreover, equality and shared power can be achieved through the mutual respect and trust built in strong working and personal relationships. Rather than glossing over these issues of power and leadership, we propose that those who work with youth address them and those who often write about the concept of "youth-leadership" honestly explore its limits across projects and institutional contexts.

## Creating Safe Spaces

As urban schools increasingly become oppressive and negative social environments for youth (Devine, 1996; Ferguson, 2001; Kozol, 1991; Kretovics & Nussel, 1993), community and city recreational programs geared for teens are phased out due to budget cuts, and public spaces such as malls ban youth through restrictive measures (Collins & Kearns, 2001; Jeffs & Smith, 1996), many youth are finding it difficult to find safe and alternative places to interact meaningfully with each other. In the projects we have worked with, special attention was paid to the need for such spaces.

For example, AYPAL recognizes the importance of creating a community environment free from the controls of schools and other public venues. Yet this CBO also realizes that such community spaces must be culturally and ethnically supportive environments where youth can build personal and leadership skills, enrich their sense of ethnic and cultural history, and gain political community organizing skills. Often in participatory research, this notion of space is addressed in terms of creating supportive venues for dialogue, such as the Highlander Center's well known method of sitting in circles in rocking chairs (Adams, 1975); however, there is less documentation on how this type of space can be created and sustained in an ethnic-specific context.

Both PARTY and TNL learned the importance of their physical meeting space. When PARTY changed their meeting venue from the sterile and "school-like" setting of a university classroom to the more comfortable and open home of one of its members, it produced a dramatic and positive shift in the ways dialogue and meetings took place, cohering the group further. Weekly PARTY meetings were a "pedagogical" space as members began reunions with a discussion of "news stories," sharing any newspaper, news magazine, or internet printout they found most salient or meaningful to their lives. These weekly discussions–the most dynamic and fruitful parts of each meeting–ultimately were used as the model when the team started teaching the government class at Jackson High. PARTY took the notion of "safe space" and dialogue into the classroom.

Likewise, TNL moved from meeting in a community center's conference room to a member's home, and later, changed the weekly meeting time from a weekday afternoon to a Saturday morning. In both cases, the changes produced positive results. Considering that middle-school and high-school youth often have very segmented days–jam packed with school, family, and work responsibilities–moving meeting times to Saturdays provided more time, less rush, and better relationship-building that not only gelled the group but improved the project's work considerably.

In all three projects, an important component of the work entailed simply creating a context appropriate space for youth to come together and dialogue other about common concerns. The lesson learned was that building and fostering these spaces is an important aspect of participatory research with youth.

### Building Trusting Relationships

Participatory research projects depend on authentic relationships and trust whether they involve adults, youth, or both (LeCompte, 1995; Maguire, 1993). Although the literature on participatory research is clear about the role of relationship-building, there is less written about how to do this specifically with *youth*, and in particularly, between youth and their adult allies. In our work with youth, we found it was critical to incorporate the youth's ways of socializing and to engage in fun activities together, to build in supports in the ways a "family" might. Here we offer some of the measures each project undertook, or had in place, to achieve this.

In AYPAL and TNL, similar ethnic and socioeconomic backgrounds of youth and adults facilitate the development of close and trusting relationships. In AYPAL, the youth frequently refer to the organization as a "family." This process of relationship-building is actively supported by AYPAL; many adult staff grew up in the same neighborhoods and attended the same public schools as the youth, allowing both parties to develop a keener understanding of each other's experiences. TNL also found that the common backgrounds of the youth and adult ally were important for creating a sense of "family" in the group.

Both TNL and PARTY found that the in-between spaces and time spent not officially meeting became as important as the work itself, such as the car drives to and from meetings, visiting each other's homes, and going to different places to eat. These non-official sites became critical places for members' reflections on the project's progress. In TNL, getting to know each other greatly informed the writing of their book because it was about their own lives as immigrants and transnationals. The TNL youth and adult ally offered each other advice and support on other milestone hurdles as well, such as college attendance, career paths, and romantic relationships. Their work demonstrates that participatory research can achieve much more than just research.

In PARTY, the group learned to be more open and flexible in carrying out the weekly meeting agenda. While PARTY members routinely and collectively developed their agendas at the start of each meeting, they discovered that when the group "strayed" from meeting items, these conversations were often the most important for learning and relationship building. Occasionally during meetings, the television or radio would be on. Rather than take away from the group's productivity, these practices helped the group develop relationships and friendships that ultimately strengthened their work together.

In all three of these projects, building relationships of trust was one of the most important aspects of the work. The lesson we learned is the importance of prioritizing relationship-building *throughout* these projects, and not to relegate it to a few "ice-breaker" activities upfront. As a result, taking the time to build and nurture relationships within the group must be prioritized as a central, not peripheral, aspect of these projects.

## CONCLUSION

This article has presented three projects and their attempts to engage youth in school, community, and social change through participatory research. As our "lessons learned" suggest, it is important to consider the ways youth identify in terms of race, class, gender, and culture, while the role of adult allies in youth-led projects should be interrogated. Additionally, the creation of safe spaces and relationships of trust are central to participatory research projects and particularly those involving urban youth. Our collective work shows that, given the opportunity, youth are capable of identifying issues and problems they face in their communities and lives; the youth in PARTY, TNL, and AYPAL are active participants in social change.

It is important to create more opportunities for meaningful youth political engagement. In a time when public schools and other public institutions routinely fail to meet the needs of urban youth, we cannot rely solely on the generosity of policy-makers or the expertise of academics and professionals to make changes in the lives of these youth. We must also draw on the vital resources, knowledge, and talents that are already present within these communities. Urban youth are consistently portrayed as disengaged, apathetic, and deficient. These prevailing images serve, in many ways, to justify the persistent social inequality and marginalization that these youth experience and to stifle possible efforts to engage the power of urban youth in meaningful projects for social change. We believe it is important not only to build more such efforts, but also to maintain a scholarly dialogue on this topic. Such a dialogue can encourage and strengthen future youth-driven projects while challenging popular representations of urban youth.

As university-based researchers who recognize our own privileged positions, we hope to spark continued discussion and exploration of ways we can do research *with* communities rather than *on* them. We may consider ourselves to be organic adult allies, but we also recognize we have one foot in the academy as researchers. Our ultimate hope is to bridge academia with community and to push academic research to be more democratic, meaningful, and of service to traditionally underserved communities. One way we have tried to practice these ideals is through participatory research: projects that combine our scholarly research with active engagement in local projects for school and community change. While we are encouraged by the potential of participatory research as a tool for social change, we also recognize it is not a panacea for the many barriers facing marginalized communities. Participatory research is not always the "best" or most appropriate method for social science research or community change (Tannock, 2004); as Paolo Freire (1993) has written: "Participatory research is no enchanted magic wand that can be waved over the culture of silence, suddenly restoring the desperately needed voice that has been forbidden to rise and to be heard" (p. ix). Even so, we contend that participatory research can be powerful. As we have seen in the work of PARTY, TNL, and AYPAL, change was effected not only in the youth's schools, homes, and communities, but also for the participants themselves–youth and adults alike.

# NOTES

1. We recognize that "youth" and "adult" are socially-constructed categories whose boundaries are constantly negotiated and shifting. For many purposes, the youth participants in these three projects (ages 13-21) would be considered "adults" and for other purposes we (ages 27-33) would be considered "youth." However, in the context of this article, we have categorized ourselves as adults, due to our institutional relationships to the other participants as their former classroom teacher, school-sanctioned mentor, volunteer staff, and university-based researchers. We also categorize the other participants as youth in part because that is how they define themselves and how they are defined by others in the various contexts of each of these projects.

2. A pseudonym.

3. Each project description is written in the first-person by the corresponding author.

4. Participants' ages correspond to the start of the project.

5. Participants' ages correspond to the start of the project.

# REFERENCES

Adams, F. (1975). *Unearthing seeds of fire: The idea of Highlander*. Winston-Salem, NC: J.F. Blair.

Ansley, F., & Gaventa, J. (1997). Researching for democracy and democratizing research. *Change*, 29, 46-53.

Anyon, J. (1997). *Ghetto schooling: A political economy of urban educational reform*. New York: Teachers College Press.

Aronowitz, S., & Giroux, H. A. (1985). *Education under siege: The conservative, liberal and radical debate over schooling*. South Hadley, MA: Bergin & Garvey Publishers, Inc.

Checkoway, B. et al. (2003). Young people as competent citizens. *Community Development Journal*, 38(4), 298-309.

Collins, D., & Kearns, R. (2001). Under curfew and under siege? Legal geographies of young people. *Geoforum*, 32, 389-403.

Devine, J. (1996). *Maximum security: The culture of violence in inner-city schools*. Chicago: University of Chicago Press.

Fals-Borda, O., & Rahman, M.A. (1991). *Action and knowledge: Breaking the monopoly with participatory action research*. New York: Apex Press.

Ferguson, A. A. (2000). *Bad boys: Public school in the making of black masculinity*. Ann Arbor: University of Michigan Press.

Fine, M. (1991). *Framing dropouts: Notes on the politics of an urban public high school*. Albany: State University of New York Press.

Finn, J. L., & Checkoway, B. (1998). Young people as competent community builders: A challenge to social work. *Social Work*, 43(4), 335-345.

Freire, P. (1993). Foreword. In P. Park et al. (eds.), *Voices of change* (pp. ix-x). Westport: Bergin & Garvey.

Gaventa, J. (1993). The powerful, the powerless, and the experts: Knowledge struggles in an information age. In Park, P., Brydon-Miller, M., Hall, B., & Jackson, T. (eds.), *Voices of change: Participatory research in the United States and Canada.* Westport: Bergin & Garvey.

Ginwright, S., & Cammarota, J. (2002). New terrain in youth development: The promise of a social justice approach. *Social Justice,* 29(4), 82-96.

Ginwright, S., & James, T. (2002). From assets to agents of change: Social justice, organizing, and youth development. *New Directions for Youth Development,* 96, 27-46.

Hall, B. (1992). From margins to center? Development and purpose of participatory research. *The American Sociologist,* 23(4), 15-28.

_____(1993). Introduction. In Park, P., Brydon-Miller, M., Hall, B., & Jackson, T. (eds.), *Voices of change: Participatory research in the United States and Canada.* Westport: Bergin & Garvey.

Jeffs, T., & Smith, M. (1996). Getting the dirtbags off the streets: Curfews and other solutions to juvenile crime. *Youth and Policy,* 52, 1-14.

Kozol, J. (1991). *Savage inequalities: Children in America's schools.* New York: Harper Collins.

Kretovics, J., & Nussel, E. (Eds.) (1994). *Transforming urban education: Problems and possibilities for equality of educational opportunity.* Boston: Allyn and Bacon.

Laz, C. (1998). Act your age. *Sociological Forum,*13(1), 85-113.

LeCompte, M. (1995). Some notes on power, agenda, and voice: A researcher's personal evolution toward critical collaborative research. In McLaren, P. & Giarelli, J.M. (eds.), *Critical Theory and Educational Research.* New York: SUNY Press.

Maguire, P. (1987). *Doing participatory research: A feminist approach.* Amherst, MA: The Center for International Education.

Maguire, P. (1993). Challenges, contradictions, and celebrations: Attempting participatory research as a doctoral student. In Park, P., Brydon-Miller, M., Hall, B., & Jackson, T. (eds.), *Voices of change: Participatory research in the United States and Canada.* Westport: Bergin & Garvey.

Males, M. (1999). *Framing youth: Ten myths about the next generation.* Monroe: Common Courage Press.

McLaughlin, M., Irby, M., & Langman, J. (1994). *Urban sanctuaries: Neighborhood organizations in the lives and futures of inner-city youth* (1st ed.). San Francisco: Jossey-Bass Publishers.

Minkler, M., & Robertson, A. (1991). The ideology of 'age/race wars': Deconstructing a social problem. *Aging and Society,* 11, 1-22.

Noguera, P. (1996). Confronting the urban in urban school reform. *The Urban Review,* 28 (1), 1-19.

_____(2003). *City schools and the American dream: Reclaiming the promise of public education.* New York: Teachers College Press.

Oakes, J. (1985). *Keeping track: How schools structure inequality.* New Haven, CT: Yale University Press.

O'Donoghue, J., Kirshner, B., & McLaughlin, M. (2002). Introduction: Moving youth participation forward. *New Directions for Youth Development,* (96), 5-7.

Park, P. (1999). People, knowledge, and change in participatory research. *Management Learning*, 30(2),141-157.

Park, P., Brydon-Miller, M.; Hall, B., & Jackson, T. (Eds.). (1993). *Voices of change: Participatory research in the United States and Canada*. Westport, CT: Bergin & Garvey.

Payne, C. (1984). *Getting what we ask for: The ambiguity of success and failure of urban education*. Westport, CT: Greenwood Press.

Tandon, R. (1981). Participatory research in the empowerment of people. *Convergence*, 14(3), 20-28.

Tannock, S. (2004). Exploring the limits of Participatory Research in Social Change. Unpublished paper.

Vio Grossi, F. (1981). Socio-political implications of participatory research. *Convergence*, 14(3), 43-50.

Youniss, J., Bales, S., Christmas-Best, V., Diversi, M., McLaughlin, M., & Silbereisen, R. (2002). Youth civic Engagement in the twenty-first century. *Journal of Research on Adolescence*, 12(1), 121-148.

Youniss, J., McLellan, J., & Yates, M. (1997). What we know about engendering civic identity. *The American Behavioral Scientist*, 40(5), 620-631.

# Youth Action for Health
# Through Youth-Led Research

Ahna Ballonoff Suleiman, MPH
Samira Soleimanpour, MPH
Jonathan London, PhD

**SUMMARY.** Youth participation in social action can contribute to healthier, more just communities and more effective youth serving institutions. Reflecting on youth-led research projects conducted in seven school-based health centers, this article presents specific youth engagement strategies, the benefits of youth participation in health research, and the lessons learned for improving adolescent health and other outcomes. *[Article copies available for a fee from The Haworth Document Delivery Service: 1-800-HAWORTH. E-mail address: <docdelivery@haworthpress.com>*

---

Ahna Ballonoff Suleiman, MPH, is Program Manager with the Contra Costa County Health Services Department, 597 Center Avenue, Suite 365, Martinez, CA 94553 (E-mail: asuleiman@hsd.ccounty.us). Samira Soleimanpour, MPH, is Project Director with the Institute for Health Policy Studies, University of California, San Francisco, 3333 California Street, Suite 265, San Francisco, CA 94143 (E-mail: samira@itsa.ucsf.edu). Jonathan London, MCP, PhD, is Senior Researcher in the Department of Human and Community Development at UC Davis, One Shields Avenue, Davis, CA 95616 (E-mail:jklondon@ucdavis.edu).

The projects described in this article were supported by Grant Number R06/CCR921786 from the Centers for Disease Control and Prevention (CDC). The contents of this article are solely the responsibility of the authors and do not necessarily represent the official views of the CDC.

[Haworth co-indexing entry note]: "Youth Action for Health Through Youth-Led Research." Suleiman, Ahna Ballonoff, Samira Soleimanpour, and Jonathan London. Co-published simultaneously in *Journal of Community Practice* (The Haworth Press, Inc.) Vol. 14. No. 1/2, 2006, pp. 125-145; and: *Youth Participation and Community Change* (ed: Barry N. Checkoway, and Lorraine M. Gutiérrez) The Haworth Press, Inc., 2006, pp. 125-145. Single or multiple copies of this article are available for a fee from The Haworth Document Delivery Service [1-800-HAWORTH, 9:00 a.m. - 5:00 p.m. (EST). E-mail address: docdelivery@haworthpress.com].

KEYWORDS. Youth-led research, health equity, participatory action research, social justice, youth development, school-based health centers

Youth participation in social action can help lay the groundwork for healthier, more just communities and more effective youth serving institutions. Youth participation in social action efforts can take many forms, including youth-led research, evaluation, planning, community organizing, or policy development. Youth participation in research and evaluation is a process in which young people actively examine issues that affect their lives and make decisions to create meaningful change in their communities with respect to these issues (London, Zimmerman, & Erbstein, 2003). Through involvement in such social change efforts, youth contribute to creating health programs and services that can better meet the needs of young people while simultaneously expanding their knowledge and skills, therefore increasing their capacity to engage in more healthful decision making. This article examines the benefits of engaging youth in health research, presents specific youth engagement strategies, and analyzes and discusses experiences with a cohort of youth-led research projects aiming to improve adolescent health and other outcomes. From the reflection on this cohort, recommendations are provided for engaging youth in social action towards personal and community health.

## YOUTH PARTICIPATION IN HEALTH-FOCUSED SOCIAL ACTION PROJECTS

Increasingly, youth participation is viewed as a vehicle for strengthening young people, their organizations and their communities (Irby, Ferber, & Pittman, with Tolman, & Yohalem, 2001; Flanagan & Faison, 2001, as cited in Pittman, Irby, Tolman, Yohalem, & Ferber, 2003) and has been incorporated into a variety of sectors and systems, including education (Rubin & Silva, 2003), environment (Harte, 1997), urban planning (Driskell, 2002), and social services (Movement Strategy Center, 2005). Health is another critical sector in which these efforts are increasingly emerging. Over ten years ago, the World Health

Organization (WHO) included youth in their call for community participation in health and outlined that effective adolescent health programs
require youth involvement in setting program objectives, policy development, and the allocation of resources at the local, national and international level (World Health Organization, 1993). This call for youth
involvement still remains crucial in light of the current health status of
youth, especially youth of color; low-income youth; immigrant youth;
lesbian, gay, bisexual, transgender, questioning, and queer youth; and
other disenfranchised groups. These youth are underserved by health
and social services and are at high risk for suicide, substance abuse and
negative sexual health outcomes (Earls, 2003; Advocates for Youth,
2004).

Substance use, pregnancy, violence, sexual transmitted infections,
asthma, and obesity only begin the long list of health challenges that
youth encounter. The most important determinants of these, and all
health issues, are related to how equitably societal and community institutions are organized and how resources are distributed (Raphael,
2003). These health issues are rooted in social inequity around income,
housing, employment opportunities, educational attainment, environment, race, and gender. Elimination of health disparities for youth can
be better achieved if young people are fully engaged as partners and
leaders in addressing social inequities, researching health issues, and
planning and evaluating health programs. Yet, to meaningfully participate in social action, young people and their communities must have the
skills necessary to address disparities in health, income, race/ethnicity,
and educational attainment (Raphael, 2003).

The approach of youth development has been an important first step
towards recognizing and building on youth as assets and authentically
engaging youth in health improvement (National Research Council &
Institute of Medicine, 2002). Youth development entails "building supports for young people and creating the opportunities for growth, learning, and exploration that are central to preparing youth for adulthood"
(Ginwright, 2003, p. 3). Yet, while youth development recognizes the
potential of youth participation in building healthier communities, it often lacks a framework that promotes and critically frames youth action
(Quiroz-Martínez, HoSang, & Villarosa, 2004). To truly create social
action, young people must have a sense of power to achieve change and
understand the context of their community (Minkler & Wallerstein,
1997). Recent theorizing has opened the way towards "social justice
youth development" as a strategy to engage youth in creating social action towards health (Ginwright & Cammarota, 2002; Ginwright, 2003;

Ginwright & James, 2003). This approach moves beyond recognizing that youth are valuable community resources capable of developing into strong adults and embraces them as powerful catalysts for community change. In social justice youth development, youth travel on a journey of self-awareness, social awareness and global awareness so that they can become powerful change agents (Ginwright & Cammarota, 2002). As youth move through these fields of awareness, they must possess strong skills to support them in collecting information, evaluating current situations, and planning for, initiating and maintaining future change.

Community-based participatory research (CBPR) is increasingly recognized as an effective strategy to eliminate health disparities, promote community change, and improve health indicators (Minkler & Wallerstein, 2003). According to Raphael (2003), the knowledge that community members possess about health and its determinants are equal to or greater than the value of experts. This concept can be applied specifically to young people. Providing young people with tools through CBPR supports them in framing their expertise so that it is integrated into overall community change. Involving youth in shaping services and programs to address health increases their sense of power and their control over and sense of responsibility for their own health (Meucci & Schwab, 1997; Schensul, 1988). As youth and adults take their power and gain mastery over their lives and their social and political environment, they can improve equity and their quality of life (Minkler & Wallerstein, 1997). Yet, neither adults nor youth can accomplish this lofty task alone. To impact the broad determinants of health, young people, as important community members, must come together and partner with adults to achieve cohesion, community participation, and political action (Raphael, 1998).

While CBPR can provide an avenue for young people to have voice in shifting health inequities, it can lack the power, on its own, to create sustainable change. When engaged as part of a cycle that integrates research, evaluation, planning, implementation, youth organizing, youth-led policy development and other social action models, a comprehensive strategy emerges. This complete cycle moves youth-led research from an academic exercise into a social action process.

Clearly, achieving social change is a long, complex process. A project that supports young people in only understanding the causes or impacts of a specific health issue will not necessarily support them in understanding or impacting the root causes of health inequity. Nor will it actually support them in developing youth-informed solutions that reflect their unique expertise. Youth-led social action efforts provide a method for youth to become empowered and to create change around these issues. As young people build their skills through youth-led research, planning, implementation and evaluation and identify important health issues in their community, they expand their knowledge and skills. As they learn the context of these health issues and explore how they are tied to the social determinants of health, including but not limited to employment, transportation, education, crime, racial inequity, poverty, and political equality, they begin to uncover the need, and potential methods, for systemic social change (Meucci & Schwab, 1997). As they present their results and begin thinking about action, the young people and their adult partners begin to strategize about how to move their information into action.

Growing evidence suggests that young people who take active roles in organizations and communities have fewer problems, are better skilled and tend to be lifelong citizens (Irby et al., 2001). Involving youth in the struggle to create social change to achieve health equity validates youths' ability to assess their needs and strengths and solve problems (Minkler, 2000). As stated by Syme (2000), individuals who are involved in social action strengthen their identity as community members, expand their skills, and learn more about their own health status which can result in health behavior change, increased locus of control over health decisions, increased empowerment, and overall better health outcomes. This notion also applies to young people. Through involvement in social change, youth channel their unique experiences and insights resulting in meaningful health reforms and more healthful delivery systems that better serve young people. Consequently, the youth participating in social action efforts also have the great potential to become local health promoters in the communities and on the issues in which they are working (Syme, 2000).

While improving the health status of the youth themselves, youth-led health research projects simultaneously benefit the community and the youth serving programs. Existing research suggests that by actively involving service recipients in planning and evaluation, the empowering process results in more effective programs (Wallerstein, 1999; Wallerstein, 2000). This concept can be applied specifically to adolescent health programs. Table 1 summarizes the benefits of engaging youth in youth-led action research that focuses specifically on health.

TABLE 1. Benefits of Engaging Youth in a Youth-Led Health Research, Social Action Framework

| Skill Building | Understanding Community Context | Action | Potential Health Outcomes |
|---|---|---|---|
| • Research<br>• Planning<br>• Implementation<br>• Evaluation<br>• Understanding of public health | • Housing<br>• Employment<br>• Poverty<br>• Transportation<br>• Education<br>• Service delivery<br>• Crime<br>• Air and water quality<br>• Institutional racism<br>• Political/social equality | • Build partnerships with other youth and adult allies<br>• Analyzing, contesting and building power<br>• Community participation<br>• Political action<br>• Problem solving | Individual level:<br>• Improved quality of life<br>• Increased locus of control<br>• Self-efficacy<br>• Self-empowerment<br>• More informed and effective health promoters<br>Community level:<br>• Improved quality of and access to services<br>• Reduced health inequities |

## The Youth Rep Approach (Youth in Focus)

Youth in Focus is a non-profit, intermediary organization based in Northern California, that provides technical assistance and training to underrepresented youth and the communities and institutions that serve them to support them in conducting Youth-Led Action Research, Evaluation and Planning (Youth REP) as a vehicle for social justice. In 2000, after more than a decade of implementing and refining youth-led action research both domestically and internationally, Youth in Focus standardized the Youth REP training process into an eight-step curriculum, called Stepping Stones, which includes youth training, adult facilitator coaching, and institutional or community capacity building. The eight-step curriculum moves youth and adult allies from an awareness of the need to engage young people as change agents into the process of building skills through Youth REP, and culminates in the boost towards action as the project comes to a close (London, 2001).[1] While the Youth REP process culminates as the action phase begins, one of Youth in Focus's key strategies is to build the capacity of youth leaders, communities and institutions to create alliances to support an effective action phase. Youth in Focus applies the Youth REP process in the fields of education, juvenile justice, community development, and adolescent public health. This paper focuses on the application of Youth REP in Youth in Focus's Adolescent Health Initiative.[2]

Youth in Focus's Adolescent Health Initiative (AHI) combines the proven tools of community-based participatory research and capacity building to engage young people in working towards health equity and social justice. The AHI works to achieve a true partnership towards health equity by bringing the science of research, evaluation and planning to the table where youth and their communities sit, so that young people can create sustainable, equitable change. The AHI supports youth and their communities in increasing their capacity to understand public health issues and to address the injustices and inequities they face by using the resources and assets they possess. Through these efforts, the AHI builds the foundation for the attainment of true health equity by creating individuals and communities primed to work towards social justice and to provide critical input on health education, promotion, service delivery and policy. As young people build their skills in Youth REP, they engage in powerful partnerships with adults and work towards achieving just, democratic, and sustainable social change.

## CASE STUDY–DOES YOUTH REP LEAD TO SOCIAL ACTION?

During the 2003-2004 school year, the University of California, San Francisco's Institute for Health Policy Studies (UCSF) contracted with Youth in Focus to implement the Youth REP Stepping Stones Curriculum at seven school based health centers (SBHCs) located in Alameda County. Each of these centers is a member of the Alameda County School Based Health Center (SBHC) Coalition. Since 1997, UCSF has conducted a comprehensive process and outcome evaluation of the Alameda County SBHC Coalition. The SBHC evaluation aims to determine how well SBHCs are serving students in Alameda County and to help SBHCs improve their programming to serve the needs of youth in their communities. In 2002, UCSF received a Community-Based Participatory Prevention Grant from the Centers for Disease Control and Prevention (CDC) to enhance their ongoing evaluation of SBHCs in Alameda County by launching a participatory student research project. The overall goals of these "Student Research Team" projects were to increase the capacity of SBHC staff and youth to engage in research on student health and to improve the quality and breadth of services offered by the SBHCs. UCSF and Youth in Focus partnered to provide support to each of the seven sites. UCSF worked with the SBHCs to coordinate and implement the logistical aspects of the projects; secured the review and approval of each site's research tools by UCSF's Internal Review Board to ensure that research procedures were conducted ethically; and provided an overview of evaluation data to each of the teams at the onset of their projects to help set the context for their research. Youth in Focus provided technical assistance and training on youth-led research to the youth and provided ongoing coaching to the primary adult facilitators on implementing the Stepping Stones Curriculum.

The youth-led projects took seven to eight months to progress through the Stepping Stones process. The youth met with a primary adult facilitator from the host site a minimum of once each week during a pre-designated meeting time, for one to two hours. They met bi-weekly or monthly with Youth in Focus staff for ongoing training in the Stepping Stones, including sessions on topic selection, research methods, data collection strategies, tool development, data analysis, and data presentation. Teams of two to six youth participated at each site and UCSF provided youth at all sites with a cash incentive to support their involvement in this project. Each team selected a health topic that they identified as important on their campus and that could be impacted by the SBHC. The teams used different strategies to identify these research topics. Several teams brainstormed within their groups to assemble a list of health topics that most significantly impacted their peers and through discussion and/or a voting process decided which topic they would research. Other teams conducted a brief needs assessment on campus to identify the largest health concerns at their schools. The health topics that the teams ultimately selected included depression, suicide, condom accessibility, birth control availability, sexual harassment, and the impact of relationships on health decision making. By the end of the school year, each of the groups had collected data on their respective topics, analyzed their data, developed recommendations based on their findings, created a final product or report, and presented their findings to key stakeholders including . the SBHC staff, school staff, community health providers, and/or community members.

These projects set out to enhance the SBHC program planning and evaluation efforts by incorporating youth voice; to identify and address health needs of the student and school community to improve the overall health and well-being of youth; and most importantly, to provide youth with a meaningful opportunity to gain valuable skills in health research, evaluation, leadership and public speaking. Although the immediate goal of these projects was not to engage participants in social action in the time period in which these projects were implemented, the question still remains: how well did these projects result in equipping youth with the necessary tools to create meaningful, sustainable social change? Perhaps the answer will take more time to emerge but this question merits further examination to assess the effectiveness of Youth REP as a social action tool.

## Case Study Methods

The following in-depth case method analyzes and discusses several key themes that arose during the implementation of youth-led research projects at seven school sites. These themes emerged through collaborative reflection by Youth in Focus and UCSF staff on their experiences with providing technical assistance to these projects and through discussions with the adult project facilitators. The discussions with the adult facilitators occurred primarily during technical assistance sessions, as well as during monthly meetings, coordinated by UCSF and Youth in Focus, which were designed to provide a forum for the facilitators to share their successes, challenges and suggestions for improvement. Further information was gathered through ongoing session reflections with the adult staff and student research team members; structured, individual interviews with each site facilitator at the end of the projects (n = 5); and student researcher pre/post surveys (n = 26).[3] The purpose of the facilitator interviews and student researcher pre/post surveys was to assess participants' experiences with the project. This analysis and reflection of the key themes helps to focus the examination of whether Youth REP can effectively lead to social action.

## Project Analysis and Discussion

### Setting the Terms for Change

One of the initial, important steps in the Youth REP process is to define the types and degrees of decision making power at each point in the process. London (2002) observes that there are two dimensions of youth decision-making in such projects: "authority" (autonomy of decisions) and "inclusion" (number of decisions). Prior to recruiting youth into the projects, the adult staff defined where the projects were to lie on these dimensions and worked to answer questions such as: do the youth have complete autonomy in selecting the project topic? If not, what restrictions or limitations are placed on topic selection? Who will work with the youth so that they understand the purpose of these limitations without feeling like pawns in the adult structure? If the adults at a site have been trying unsuccessfully to achieve change in a specific area, does it make sense for the youth to engage in impacting the same topic? If there are multiple levels of stakeholders (i.e., program staff, school administrators, the school board, community health providers), who should be involved from the beginning in shaping the focus of the project? Resolving these questions during the initial phases of the project allowed the projects to move forward as smoothly as possible (see Table 2).

Despite work to answer these questions early on in these projects, the answers often changed mid-stream and new questions continually arose. For example, at one site the SBHC staff and the school principal originally supported a project looking at condom accessibility among students, but when the Youth REP participants returned to the principal to begin data collection, they were informed that students would need parental consent before participating in their research and later learned that many teachers and parents were strongly opposed to research on this topic. At another site, the youth team initially elected to research better ways to market the SBHC services to the student body. They quickly learned that the SBHC was already operating close to capacity and would not be able to respond to a sudden flood of new clients. Considering that it often took three to four weeks for groups to agree on a topic, having to go back to the drawing board for topic selection seemed insurmountable. What happens at this point? Do the youth, who are already working on a short timeline, return to the drawing board to select another topic? Do the adults who supported this topic advocate for the youth? While the second option is preferable, at times the adults lack the power to influence those in opposition or may have political or personal reasons not to push the agenda of the youth researchers. When the first option occurs, this can often have devastating impacts on the morale and commitment of the youth participants. In the first example above, the youth remained committed to their topic and shifted their timeline to accommodate the need for parental consent. In the second case, the

TABLE 2. Setting the Terms for Change

| | |
|---|---|
| 1. | Define types and levels of decision making power between youth and adults. |
| 2. | Ensure that all partners are aware of agreements for making decisions and provide clear, thorough explanations to youth and adults when these agreements change. |
| 3. | Prepare adults to serve as allies for youth. |
| 4. | Prepare youth for the slow pace and potential challenges of social change. |

youth returned to the drawing board and selected a new topic. Due to the solid collaborative relationship between the youth and adults at this site, this shift required some adjustment to the timeline, but resulted in both the youth and the adults feeling positive about the future of the project.

In addition to setting the agenda for change, it is important for the adult stakeholders to truly understand youth leadership and their role as allies. The youth process often takes longer and is much less linear than adults are used to experiencing. A strong adult ally helps create space and structure to allow for this process but does not jump into problem solving or directing the youth team. This can often be frustrating for adults, especially when they have an agenda they feel is particularly important. During the beginning of the project, the adults must be coached to loosen their grip on their personal agendas and prepare for the creative process of the youth team. As one of the site coordinators in this cohort reflected, "The process felt totally youth-led and it has changed my teaching style a lot. I just throw every question back at them now. They know the answers. Youth leadership is the coolest part of this project–that's also why it takes so long." The adults in the project must build their skills to support the youth teams without dictating the direction.

To prepare young people for these types of challenges, part of the context building that happens early on in the projects includes an examination of existing power structures and the cycle of social and institutional change. Young people must understand that change can be challenging and often controversial, even when it is moving towards something better. In addition, they must be grounded in the idea that change often comes with a high price, which may include losing a job, jeopardizing program funding, or creating controversy and division among key allies. The more that young people understand the realities and context of social action, the better prepared they will be to anticipate and negotiate the challenges that arise in their projects.

## Sustaining Youth Engagement

Rarely does institutional and community change happen quickly and maintaining youth engagement through the ups and downs of the change cycle can be challenging. Young people have many things competing for their attention. The fast pace of today's world now requires even more effort to engage youth in consistent, ongoing activities. With the slow pace of social change, how do we keep young people engaged?

The slow cycle of change can often result in low morale at various points in a Youth REP project. In these projects, interest and enthusiasm started out high as the young people began to think about action. They wanted to dive into creating change and worry about collecting data later. To harness this enthusiasm, each group developed a concept map for the change they hoped to see in their projects. The maps outlined the problem each group wanted to address, the information they wanted to collect, and the change that they wanted to see as a result of their work. The youth looking at condom accessibility wanted to see condoms available in their school-based health centers so that there were fewer pregnancies and sexually transmitted infections on campus. The youth looking at depression wanted the school and community to have a more integrated approach to youth depression so that more services were available and there was less stigma among young people around mental health. One facilitator posted her group's map in her office and often pulled it out for meetings and as the shape of the project changed, so did the shape of the group's map. These maps helped each group shape a vision for the year. The groups that held the clearest vision for change appeared more engaged throughout the project.

In addition to a clear vision, youth must have multiple opportunities to present and obtain feedback on their process and their data. One of the most exciting times in the projects occurred when the youth began their data collection process. After months of working through selecting a topic, defining a research question, and developing data collection tools, the youth finally had the opportunity to share with others the work they were doing. As they collected their data they heard feedback from their peers and adults about the importance of the topic they had selected. One team fielded questions from school administrators, parents and students when they presented their topic of condom accessibility at a school health fair. They engaged in discussions with people who both strongly supported and opposed increasing student access to condoms on campus. This opportunity allowed the students to clarify their own opinions and better understand opposing views. As the groups gathered more suggestions about how to address the issues they were examining, they began to expand their vision for social action. As they began to collect data, the topic each group had selected began to take shape for the larger school community. Most importantly, the youth researchers repeatedly faced the question, "So what are you going to do with all of this information once you are done?" Their immediate answer to this question was that they would analyze the data they collected. The longer-term and more compelling answer that began to emerge was that they wanted to take the information they collected to initiate significant change in the institutions designed to serve them and in their communities as a whole. Throughout the Youth REP process, youth must be supported to remember and work from their vision for change.

But often the vision is not enough–the youth must also have the opportunity to experience social action during the process of the project. For example, one group of researchers had become very disengaged as their Youth REP project neared the end. The adults tried countless strategies to keep the youth engaged by providing opportunities for them to present at local conferences, integrating team building activities into their regular meetings, providing outreach to the youth individually to see what they needed to reengage–all with limited success. The youth would show up variably and apathy during meetings was high. Despite the apathy, the group was able to pull through, complete their data collection and present their findings to a group of community health providers, city health officials, and school-based health center providers. During this presentation, the city health officials responded enthusiastically to the data the youth had collected and the recommendations they had made. The officials made suggestions that this data should be shared with the school board, the mayor and other key community stakeholders. They also felt that this information should be presented to adolescent health providers throughout the country. In that moment, the group of youth who could barely be convinced to show up for a meeting a week prior were suddenly committing to working on the project for another school year and meeting over the summer. This positive reflection from key stakeholders outside of the project provided a critical context to sustain the engagement of these young people. The change now extended beyond their work and seemed to have connection with something larger. Integrating opportunities to connect with the larger context and larger social action movements throughout the project is key for sustained youth involvement.

## Creating a Realistic Timeline

One of the primary challenges of working with young people in school-based projects is the limitation of the academic calendar. During the initial months of school, students are learning new schedules, making decisions about extra-curricular activities and often acclimating to a new school environment. Although this cohort aimed to get the Youth REP projects running in September, most of the projects were not underway until October and some start-dates lingered into November.

This was due to both limitations from the youth and the adults in the project. The adults were frequently overloaded with beginning of the year meetings, programs and activities. The youth were often making decisions between participating in this project versus participating in a sport, band or securing an after school job to supplement their families' incomes. Even in sites committed to an early start, some attrition occurred during the first two months as youth made tough decisions about how to spend their time (see Table 3).

This challenge of time was further enhanced when breaks, holidays, testing and other items on the academic calendar resulted in cancelled meetings or youth unable or unwilling to attend scheduled meetings. For example, during the months of January and February when three school holidays (Dr. Martin Luther King Jr.'s Day, Lincoln's Birthday, and Washington's Birthday) and first semester finals occurred, groups scheduled to meet on Mondays lost four meeting times in a period of six weeks. While attempts were made to reschedule these meetings, it was often challenging to coordinate the schedules of up to six busy youth, one adult facilitator, and facilities that are already overbooked. During these challenging times, the timeline for the Youth REP project was continually revised and the groups struggled to stay involved and engaged in the process.

Due to these challenges with timing, although all groups were scheduled to complete their research process and begin their action phase during the month of May, everyone was scrambling to complete their research and engage in small action steps as the school year ended in June. Although many of the groups delivered powerful presentations where the seeds were laid for significant social and programmatic change, none of the groups were able to engage in achieving this change during the school year. Several of the groups were interested in continuing work on their projects to achieve social action, however, they will not be able to re-convene as a whole next year due to the fact that they

TABLE 3. Sustaining Youth Engagement

1.  Support youth in creating a clear vision and timeline for the full scope of the project.
2.  Provide multiple opportunities for youth throughout the project to present and get feedback and encouragement on their content and process.
3.  Create multiple opportunities for youth to reflect upon, engage in and initiate social action.
4.  Network with larger social action allies and movement organizations throughout the project duration to provide the "bigger picture" and support action.

lost members to graduation or school transfers. One site lost their entire group to graduation and another lost all but one member. Three of the groups have committed to continuing work on the social action portions of their projects next year and the host sites are all working to allocate staff and resources to support those young people.

One solution to these challenges with the timeline is scheduling youth-led action research projects on a two year cycle. Although not appropriate for all settings, in this model, resources should be secured at the onset of the project to support a two year process and youth should be recruited who are not slated for graduation for a minimum of two years. When youth are recruited, they should understand that they are engaging in a two year process with the first year focusing on Youth REP and the second year focusing on action. To support the social action component, early alliances should be formed with individuals and institutions that can support the youth in organizing, policy development, and ongoing research. In addition, timelines should be set out to match the specific academic calendar for each school site so that the actual number of meetings young people are able to attend matches the scope of work they lay out for themselves (see Table 4).

## Towards Social Action

Each of the projects in this cohort resulted in some type of change, either at the individual, group, community and/or institutional level. The youth were engaged in a powerful year-long process that built their understanding of a critical health issue; their research and public speaking skills; and their sense of self-efficacy. After participating in this project, students reported that they better understood how to create a research tool (100%, n = 26) and a research paper (96%, n = 25) and felt more like leaders (92%, n = 24). Using a "think globally, act locally" model of change, these individual skills have great potential to help youth engage in social action both now and in the future. Youth in Focus's social change model that guided the projects can be summarized in Figure 1, which presents a nested understanding of the factors that can lead to increases in youth agency.

At the core of the model are self-beliefs, most importantly a sense of self-efficacy (Bandura 1977, 1989). Without such understandings of self, none of the other subsequent factors can take hold. Content knowledge, in this case adolescent health issues, allows for informed action. Skills, in this case youth-led action research, evaluation, and planning, provide the tools needed to gather, analyze, and apply knowledge. An

TABLE 4. Creating a Realistic Timeline

1.  Begin as early as possible.

2.  Plan backwards from the ultimate goal.

3.  Consider a two year project cycle.

4.  From the onset, set realistic and inspiring goals for the project.

5.  Examine potential scheduling conflicts and create a schedule with the least possible interruption, with high activity project periods occurring during less demanding times in the academic year whenever possible.

FIGURE 1. Youth Agency for Social Change Model

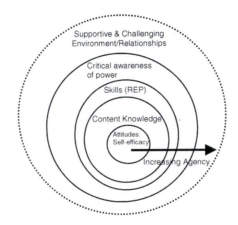

awareness of power sets these self-beliefs, knowledge and skills in a critical context, allowing youth to understand their own experience as shaping and shaped by broader social, political, cultural, and historical patterns. Finally, the project environment, a product of relationships with the facilitator, peers, and the surrounding organization offers a supportive forum in which to experiment, grow, and act (Zeldin, Camino & Mook, 2005). All of these factors are necessary to enable the development and the enactment of youth agency for effective social change.

The student research projects represented an initial and important attempt to implement this model. Based on the survey data, the majority of the student researchers reported increased levels of self-efficacy (73%, n = 19) after participating in this project. As described above, the projects attempted, and largely succeeded, in developing the students' content knowledge and Youth REP skills. In most cases, a supportive environment with positive youth-adult partnerships was present. The agencies the youth worked with all learned how to better listen to and integrate youth voice and support youth-led decision-making and also learned from the challenges of keeping young people engaged in this process. Because of time limitations, projects were less successful in promoting a critical analysis of power through placing the adolescent health issues in broader social, political, cultural, and historical contexts, and supporting a sense of the students as health activists. The project timelines that concluded with the production of the student research without adequate opportunities to develop and implement action plans also prevented a full version of this model from being realized. Nonetheless, the projects did achieve some notable successes.

For example, the work of the students who researched condom availability during this cohort was continued by a group of students during the 2004-2005 school year. This second group of students focused their research specifically on teen pregnancy and collected data through focus groups and interviews with parenting and non-parenting youth. The students were able to take the results of their study to the school board resulting in the revision of the school district's condom availability policy, allowing all high schools to dispense condoms and other contraceptive methods through the school based health clinics and health educators to dispense condoms during high school health education presentations. At another site, students who researched depression and suicide created a pocket-sized "Teen Resource Guide" in an effort to educate their peers and raise awareness on this topic. The guide included a brief checklist for students to assess whether they needed to talk to someone immediately about emotional health concerns, as well names and numbers of agencies that could be contacted when they are considering suicide or just feeling depressed. These guides were distributed by the health center during the 2004-2005 school year.

This illustrates how youth involvement in social change can improve decision making around issues that impact youth. At some sites, school based health center staff are looking at strategies to sustain youth involvement in service design, delivery and evaluation. In addition, several of the sites are searching for ways to provide continued support for the youth to pursue the action phase of their projects. The full impact of the change may not yet be evident and may not even be measured, but Youth in Focus, UCSF, and other partners are continuing to develop strategies to strengthen the social action impact of their projects. Beyond the initial on-the-ground impacts, these projects offer the promise of far greater social change, because of the success in transforming youth from passive recipients of health services to critical informed and active stakeholders in the production of such services and the shaping of broader institutional and policy environments that influence their health and that of their peers.

## CONCLUSION

Although the explicit focus of this cohort of projects was not to engage youth in social action, it was demonstrated that youth and their adult allies who participate in Youth REP can effectively move towards social action if key components are incorporated into the process. Specifically, the level and context of decision-making power must be transparent to all partners from the onset of the efforts. Additionally, youth should have ample opportunities to realize the purpose and value of their work so that they can feel connected to the process. Youth and their adult allies also need to create a realistic timeline to ensure that youth have sufficient time to understand the context of their work and execute their recommended strategies for action. Lastly, it is essential that all partners are committed to implementing and sustaining the action efforts initiated by youth. If these strategies are applied, a strong foundation is built for effective social action to ensue.

As demonstrated by Wallerstein (1999, 2000), by actively involving service recipients in planning and evaluation, the empowering process can result in more effective programs. The Youth REP model is designed to increase youth's understanding of health issues and enhance their skills to identify health priorities, design and implement a research project, and summarize and disseminate their research findings and recommendations. Ultimately, participation in this process empowers youth to engage in social action, in this case providing critical input into the design and delivery of health programming and policy. As the young people in these Youth REP projects developed their skills and knowledge, they were subsequently able to partner with their adult allies to create concrete improvements in the school-based health center programming.

Thus, when accompanied by strategies to push towards action, Youth REP helps young people build valuable skills for creating sustainable social change for healthier communities. Through these projects, the youth participants built their capacity as community-based researchers and ultimately social action agents, enhanced the youth directed services and programs in their SBHCs, and built essential partnerships among youth and adult stakeholders. Although the cycle of social change can be slow and complicated, and involving youth can make it feel even more complex, the potential for meaningful, healthy, sustainable change grows exponentially as youth leaders join the process.

## NOTES

1. More information on Youth In Focus can be found at www.youthinfocus.net
2. Other notable youth-led action research projects on health and equity have been conducted by the Freedom Bound Center (*http://www.freedomboundcenter.org/projects.htm*), Davis Blacks for Effective Community Action (access at *www.youthinfocus.net/ whatsnew_news.htm*), Youth United for Community Action (*http://www.youthunited.net/*), the Institute for Community Research/Youth Action Research Institute (*http://www. incommunityresearch.org/research/yari.htm*), and Communities for a Better Environment (*http://www.cbecal.org/youth/index.shtml*).
3. During the 2003-2004 school year, over 40 students initially participated in the Student Research Team project. Of these students, 28 high school and five middle school youth stayed in the program through the end of the school year. Data presented from the student researcher pre/post survey includes only high school youth who completed both a pre and a post-survey (n = 26).

## REFERENCES

Advocates for Youth. (2004, January). *The facts: Youth of color–at disproportionate risk of negative sexual health outcomes.* Retrieved May 2, 2005, from http://www.advocatesforyouth.org/publications/factsheet/fsyouthcolor.htm

Bandura, A. (1977). Self-efficacy: Toward a unifying theory of behavioral change. *Psychological Review, 84* (2), 191-215.

Bandura, A. (1989). Human agency in social cognitive theory. *American Psychologist, 44*, 1175-1184.

Driskell, D. (2002). Creating better cities with children and youth: A manual for participation. Sterling, VA: UNESCO Publishers, Management of Social Transformation (MOST).

Earls, M. (2003). The facts: GLBTQ youth: At risk and underserved. Washington, DC: Advocates for Youth.

Flanagan, C.A., & Faison, N. (2001). Youth civic development: Implications of research for social policy and programs. Social Policy Report, *15* (1). As cited in Pittman, K., Irby, M., Tolman, J., Yohalem, N., & Ferber, T. (2003). Preventing problems, promoting development, encouraging engagement: Competing priorities or inseparable goals? Washington, DC: The Forum for Youth Investment, Impact Strategies, Inc. Available online at www.forumfyi.org

Ginwright, S. (2003). Youth organizing: Expanding the possibilities for youth development. *Occasional paper series on youth organizing, No. 3.* New York: Funders Collaborative on Youth Organizing.

Ginwright, S., & James, T. (2002, Winter). From assets to agents of social change: Social justice, organizing, and youth development. *New directions in youth development, 96,* 27-46.

Ginwright, S., & Cammarota, J. (2002). New terrain in youth development: The promise of a social justice approach. *Social Justice, 9* (4), 82-95.

Hart, R. (1997). *Children's participation: The theory and practice of involving young citizens in community development and environmental care.* New York: Earthscan.

Irby, M., Ferber, T., & Pittman, K. with Tolman, J., & Yohalem, N. (2001). Youth action: Youth contributing to communities, communities supporting youth. *Community & youth development series, Vol. 6.* Takoma Park, MD: The Forum for Youth Investment, International Youth Foundation.

London, J. (2001). Youth REP: Step by step: An introduction to youth-led evaluation and research. Oakland, CA: Youth in Focus.

London, J., Zimmerman, K., & Erbstein, N. (2003). Youth-led research, evaluation and planning as youth, organizational and community development. In K. Sabo (Ed.), Youth participatory evaluation: A field in the making. *New Directions in Evaluation, 98, Special Issue,* 33-45.

Meucci, S., & Schwab, M. (1997). Children and the environment: Young people's participation in social change. *Social Justice, 24* (3), 1-10.

Minkler, M. (2000). Health promotion at the dawn of the 21st century: Challenges and dilemmas. In M. Schneider Jammer & D. Stokols (Eds.), *Promoting human wellness: New frontiers for research, practice and policy* (pp. 349-377). Berkeley, CA: University of California Press.

Minkler, M., & Wallerstein, N. (1997). Improving health through community organization and community building. In K. Glanz, F. Lewis, B. Rimer (Eds.), *Health behavior and health education: Theory, research and practice* (2nd ed., pp. 241-269). San Francisco, CA: Jossey-Bass.

Minkler, M., & Wallerstein, N. (2003). Introduction to community-based participatory research. In M. Minkler & N. Wallerstein (Eds.), *Community-based participatory research for health* (pp. 3-26). San Francisco, CA: Jossey-Bass.

Movement Strategy Center. (2005). Bringing it together: Uniting youth organizing, development and services for long-term sustainability. Oakland, CA: Movement Strategy Center.

National Research Council & Institute of Medicine. (J. Eccles & J. A. Gootman, Eds.). (2002). *Community programs to promote youth development.* Washington, DC: National Academy Press.

Pittman, K., Irby, M., Tolman, J., Yohalem, N., & Ferber, T. (2003). *Preventing problems, promoting development, encouraging engagement: Competing priorities or inseparable goals?* Washington, DC: The Forum for Youth Investment, Impact Strategies, Inc. Retrieved May 1, 2005, from www.forumfyi.org

Quiroz-Martínez, J., HoSang, D., & Villarosa, L. (2004). Changing the rules of the game: Youth development and structural racism. Washington, DC: Philanthropic Initiative for Racial Equity.

Raphael, D. (1998). Public health responses to health inequities. *Canadian Journal of Public Health, 89,* 380-381.

Raphael, D. (2003). A society in decline: The political, economic and social determinants in health inequities in the United States. In R. Hofrichter (Ed.), *Health and social justice: Politics, ideology and inequity in the distribution of disease* (pp. 59-88). San Francisco, CA: Jossey-Bass.

Rubin, B., & Silva, E. (Eds.). (2003) *Critical voices in school reform: Students living through changes.* London: Routledge.

Schensul, J. (1988). Community-based risk prevention with urban youth. *School Psychology Review, 27* (2), 233-245.

Syme, S. (2000). Community participation, empowerment and health: Development of a wellness guide for California. In M. Schneider Jammer & D. Stokols (Eds.), *Promoting human wellness: New frontiers for research, practice and policy* (pp. 78-98). Berkeley, CA: University of California Press.

Wallerstein, N. (1999, July). Power between evaluator and community: Research relationships within New Mexico's healthier communities. *Soc Sci Med, 49* (1), 39-53.

Wallerstein, N. (2000, March-June). A participatory evaluation model for healthier communities: Developing indicators for New Mexico. *Public Health Rep, 115* (2-3), 199-204.

World Health Organization. (1993). *The health of young people: A challenge and a promise.* England: Macmillan/Clays.

Zeldin, S., Camino, L., & Mook, C. (2005). The adoption of innovation in youth organizations: Creating the conditions for youth-adult partnerships. *Journal of Community Psychology, 33*(1), 121-135.

# Youth Participation in Photovoice as a Strategy for Community Change

Caroline C. Wang, DrPH, MPH

**SUMMARY.** Photovoice is a participatory action research strategy which can contribute to youth mobilization for community change. The strategy can enable youth to (1) record and vivify their community's strengths and concerns; (2) promote critical dialogue and knowledge about community issues through group discussion of photographs; and (3) reach policy makers. Following a description of the photovoice methodology, this article briefly highlights ten projects in which youth used photovoice to represent, advocate, and enhance community health and well-being. *[Article copies available for a fee from The Haworth Document Delivery Service: 1-800-HAWORTH. E-mail address: <docdelivery@ haworthpress.com> Website: <http://www.HaworthPress.com> © 2006 by The Haworth Press, Inc. All rights reserved.]*

**KEYWORDS.** Photovoice, youth participation, advocacy, photography, policy, community action

Caroline C. Wang is affiliated with the School of Public Health, University of Michigan, 1420 Washington Heights, Ann Arbor, MI 48109-2029 (E-mail: wangc@umich.edu).

[Haworth co-indexing entry note]: "Youth Participation in Photovoice as a Strategy for Community Change." Wang, Caroline C. Co-published simultaneously in *Journal of Community Practice* (The Haworth Press, Inc.) Vol. 14, No. 1/2, 2006, pp. 147-161; and: *Youth Participation and Community Change* (ed: Barry N. Checkoway, and Lorraine M. Gutiérrez) The Haworth Press, Inc., 2006, pp. 147-161. Single or multiple copies of this article are available for a fee from The Haworth Document Delivery Service [1-800-HAWORTH, 9:00 a.m. - 5:00 p.m. (EST). E-mail address: docdelivery@haworthpress.com].

doi:10.1300/J125v14n01_09

In Baltimore, Maryland, a 12-year-old photographs a six-year-old boy in a bar with a 17-year-old sister who was drinking, and writes that any young person in the neighborhood has access to a cigarette vending machine and perhaps alcohol (Strack, Magill, & McDonagh, 2003). In Flint, Michigan, a high school sophomore photographs a young, educated Black man holding a camera to illustrate how racial profiling might lead to false accusations of stealing (Tom-Quinn, 2002). And in a town in Western Australia, a 14-year-old aborigine photographs a hotel on the main street with a sign that says, "Restaurant Open. Skimpy today and tonight" and notes, "Skimpies are women walking around naked, half naked" (Larson, Mitchell, & Gilles, 2001). Living in places far afield from one another, these young persons used a methodology called "photovoice" to contribute to their community's health and well-being. Drawing from ten examples of photovoice projects in places ranging from the San Francisco Bay area to South Africa, this article discusses the contributions of the methodology as a strategy for engaging youth in policy advocacy and community change.

## PHOTOVOICE–OVERVIEW

Photovoice is a participatory action research (PAR) method based on health promotion principles and the theoretical literature on education for critical consciousness, feminist theory, and a community-based approach to documentary photography (Wang & Burris, 1997; Wang, Burris, & Xiang, 1996). Rooted in democratic ideals, the methodology entails providing people with cameras so that they can photograph their everyday realities. Photovoice is based on the concepts that images teach, pictures can influence policy, and community people ought to participate in creating and defining the images that shape healthful public policy (Wang, 1999).

The photovoice concept, method, and use for participatory action research were created by Caroline Wang and Mary Ann Burris, and applied first in the Ford Foundation-supported Women's Reproductive Health and Development Program in Yunnan, China (Wang & Burris, 1997; Wang, Burris, & Xiang, 1996; Wang, Wu, Zhan, & Carovano, 1998). Photovoice has three main goals: to enable people to (1) record and represent their everyday realities; (2) promote critical dialogue and knowledge about personal and community strengths and concerns; and (3) reach policymakers. The application of photovoice towards conducting participatory needs assessment, asset-mapping, and evaluation, as well as reaching policy makers, has been discussed elsewhere (Killion & Wang, 2000; Wang, 1999, 2003; Wang & Burris, 1997; Wang, Burris, & Xiang, 1996; Wang, Cash, & Powers, 2000; Wang & Pies, 2004; Wang, Wu, Zhan, & Carovano, 1998; Wang, Yuan, & Feng, 1996).

The purpose of this article is to take a modest step toward examining youth participation in photovoice. The article is divided into three sections. The Methods section below describes the steps developed for photovoice. Second, ten photovice projects defined by youth participation and public advocacy are briefly highlighted. Finally, in the Discussion section, contributions and limitations for youth participation in community change are discussed.

## PHOTOVOICE METHODS

A nine-step strategy to mobilize community action through the use of photovoice is presented below.

1. *Select and recruit a target audience of policy makers or community leaders.* Who has the power to make decisions that can improve the situation? The target audience may include city council members and other politicians, journalists, physicians, administrators, researchers, business people, and community leaders with the power to make and implement participants' recommendations. As an ad hoc advisory board to the project, their primary role is to serve as a group with the political will to put participants' ideas into practice. The inter-generational Flint Photovoice and other projects have created "guidance groups" of policy makers and sympathetic community leaders who serve as the influential audience for participants' images, stories, and recommendations.

2. *Recruit a group of photovoice participants.* To allow for practical ease and in-depth discussion, seven to ten people is an ideal group size. Youth photovoice participants have been recruited and mobilized through elementary, middle, and high schools, church groups, vocational programs, clinics, and teen centers. In addition, projects in which both youth and adults take photographs, such as Flint Photovoice, provide an opportunity to gain comparative generational perspectives on community issues. It should be noted that step 1 and step 2 are interchangeable in sequence; youth

participants could come together first and then decide upon their primary intended audience/s.

3. *Introduce the photovoice methodology to participants, and facilitate a group discussion about cameras, power, and ethics.* The first workshop begins with an introduction to the photovoice concept and method. It emphasizes the aim to influence policy makers and community leaders; the responsibility and authority conferred upon the photographer wielding the camera; an ethic of giving photographs back to community people to express thanks; and how to minimize potential risks to youth participants' well-being. To support this last point, facilitators and youth photographers discuss questions that include:

- What is an acceptable way to approach someone to take their picture?
- Whether you ought to take pictures of other people without their knowledge?
- When would you *not* want to have your picture taken?
- To whom might you wish to give photographs, and what might be the implications?

4. *Obtain informed consent.* One hallmark of photovoice training is that the first session emphasizes safety and the authority and responsibility that come with using a camera. Facilitators must consider how participants' vulnerability may be further modified by their young age, as well as their social class, access to power (or lack thereof), health concerns, and other factors. Facilitators should explain the written informed consent form, which ought to include a statement of project activities and significance, specific potential risks and benefits, the voluntary nature of participation and freedom to withdraw at any time for any reason, and the understanding that no photographs identifying specific individuals will be released without separate written consent of not only the photographer but also the identified individuals (Wang & Redwood-Jones, 2001). The informed consent of parents or guardians for all minors, as well as youth participants' consent, must be obtained.

5. *Pose initial theme/s for taking pictures.* Participants may wish to brainstorm together about what themes they can focus upon to enhance community health, and then determine individually what

they wish to photograph. Or, given a specific project theme such as violence prevention, participants may discuss ways in which they might portray conditions and factors that contribute to or prevent violence. For subsequent rounds of picture-taking, participants can generate specific, related ways of thinking about what to photograph in terms of open-ended questions.

6. *Distribute cameras to participants and review how to use the camera.* What kind of camera should be used? At least four different kinds of cameras have been used for photovoice projects: autofocus, autorewind cameras; disposable cameras; medium format Holga cameras; and digital cameras. The choice of camera can be guided by facilitators' and participants' preferences and practical considerations. For example, if participants will take more than two or three rolls of film, then disposable cameras may be least cost-effective. If participants have a strong interest in using a camera that allows for maximum creative expression, and facilitators are experienced with the medium format Holga, then they may prefer this inexpensive camera that permits multiple exposures so that people can literally layer the meaning of their images.

7. *Provide time for participants to take pictures.* Participants agree to turn in their images to a facilitator for developing and/or enlarging at a specified time, such as one week after the initial workshop, and then to gather again to discuss their photographs.

8. *Meet to discuss photographs and identify themes.* The next three stages–selecting photographs, contextualizing or storytelling, and codifying issues, themes, or theories–occur during group discussion. First, each participant may be asked to select and talk about one or two photographs that s/he feels is most significant, or simply likes best. Second, participants may frame stories about–and take a critical stance toward–their photographs in terms of questions spelling the mnemonic SHOWeD:

- What do you *S*ee here?
- What's really *H*appening here?
- How does this relate to *O*ur lives?
- *W*hy does this situation, concern, or strength exist?
- What can we *D*o about it?

Third, participants codify the issues, themes, or theories that arise from their photographs. Given that photovoice is well-suited to action-oriented analysis that creates practical guidelines, participants may particularly focus on issues. These stages are carried out for each round of photographs taken by participants. The number of photovoice rounds will depend on factors that include facilitators' and participants' preferences, overall project scope and budget, and other practical considerations. One to six rounds were carried out for most of the photovoice projects discussed in this paper.

9. *Plan with participants a format to share photographs and stories with policy makers or community leaders.* Facilitators and participants typically plan a format such as a Powerpoint slide show or an exhibition to amplify participants' photographs, stories, and recommendations to policy makers and community leaders. For example, in Flint Photovoice, facilitators and participants organized a slide show and exhibition held at the city's main library where youth and adult participants shared their photographs and stories with an audience that included the mayor, journalists, community leaders, and researchers.

The above outline provides a brief methodological overview. A detailed discussion of photovoice methodology can be found in Wang and Burris (1997) and Wang and Redwood-Jones (2001).

## PHOTOVOICE PROJECTS WITH YOUTH PARTICIPATION FOR COMMUNITY ACTION

As the Editors of this volume note, youth participation "expresses the view of youth as competent citizens and active participants in the institutions and decisions that affect their lives." Photovoice offers an ideal way for young people to harness the power of these roles to enhance their community's well-being. Innovative photovoice projects grounded in youth participation and youth culture have been initiated around the US and the world; it is beyond the scope of this paper to offer a comprehensive review of all such projects. Ten projects known to the author, summarized in Table 1 and described briefly below, provide examples of intergenerational photovoice initiatives that promote youth participation and community change.

*Youth Against Violence Photovoice.* This project brought together young people from around Flint to generate photographs and dialogue

TABLE 1. Intergenerational Photovoice to Promote Youth Participation and Community Change

| Project Title Location | Funding Source | Theme of Project | Participants Who Took Photographs | Primary Intended Audience |
|---|---|---|---|---|
| Youth Against Violence Photovoice Flint, Michigan | Centers for Disease Control and Prevention | Conditions that contribute to or prevent violence | Elementary through high school youth | Community Steering Committee and community members |
| Photovoice Youth Empowerment Program Clarkston, Georgia | DeKalb County Board of Health; Kenneth Cole Foundation | Community health issues and concerns | African American and refugee high school students | Clarkston Boards of Health and Education, Clarkston officials, law enforcement officers and the business community |
| Town Criers Photovoice Oakland, California | California Wellness Foundation | AIDS epidemic among African Americans | Black and Latino youth who knew someone infected with HIV or AIDS | Mainstream and ethnic media |
| Flint Photovoice Flint, Michigan | Charles Stewart Mott Foundation | Assets and issues exerting the greatest impact on individual and community health and well-being | Youth participants in the National Institute for Drug Abuse-supported Flint Adolescent Study; youth active in community leadership roles; adult neighborhood activists; and local policy makers and community leaders | Policy makers and community leaders |
| Youth Empowerment Strategies! Oakland, California | Centers for Disease Control & Prevention | Concerns and issues that can be targeted for social action | Fifth graders attending public elementary Title I schools serving low income communities | School principals, after-school coordinators, and teachers |
| Picture Me Tobacco Free: A Youth Photovoice Action Project North Carolina | State's tobacco settlement funds | Influence of tobacco within young people's lives and communities | Youth from African American Baptist churches | Local church leaders, churchgoers, and community members |
| Youth Photovoice Baltimore, Maryland | Johns Hopkins University Center for Adolescent Health/ Centers for Disease Control & Prevention | Community assets and deficits | Adolescents involved in an afterschool teen center | Policy makers, researchers, and community leaders |
| Teen Photovoice: An Educational Empowerment Program Los Angeles, California | Robert Wood Johnson Clinical Scholars Program | Influences upon their health behaviors | Minority high school students serving on a Youth Advisory Council for the UCLA/RAND Center for Adolescent Health Promotion | Mainstream media and researchers at the UCLA/RAND Center for Adolescent Health Promotion |
| Photovoice for Tobacco, Drug, and Alcohol Prevention Among Adolescents Western Cape, South Africa | National Cancer Institute/Fogarty International Center | What is important in their lives, and who is important in their lives | Young people in three racially diverse high schools | Health researchers and policy makers |
| Young Aboriginal People's View of Sexual Health Carnarvon, Western Australia | Health Department of Western Australia | What young local people think about HIV, in what ways local Aboriginal youth are protected from HIV, and what are the reasons young people may be at risk | Aboriginal youth | Health Department staff |

about their experiences and perceptions of the root causes and solutions to violence in their communities. Teen participants brought in photographs of people and discussed negative attitudes, such as how hard it is deal with anger or resist the fun of a play fight. Older teen participants took more metaphorical pictures to illustrate important positive attitudes that work against violence such as freedom from stereotypes and peer pressure. Several took images to represent prejudice as a cause of violence. Through a civic participation component called KidSpeak, students presented testimony directly to a panel of city council members, county commissioners, state legislators and other policy makers. The project signified a critical coalescence of youth activism, creativity, and leadership to give youth a voice in developing violence prevention policies and programs (Morrel-Samuels, Wang, Bell, & Monk, 2005).

*Photovoice Youth Empowerment Program.* The DeKalb County Board of Health recruited and hired 50 high school students to participate in this program for three of four recent summers. One-third of the students were African American and the others were from refugee families. The students sought to reach leaders in the Clarkston policy, education, law enforcement, and business community. Participants reported acquiring computer and presentation skills, developing self-confidence, and learning to work with those different from themselves. The city's mayor has started a recycling program catalyzed by student presentations and recommendations (Cottrell, 2005).

*Town Criers Photovoice.* Alameda County, California, was the first U.S. county to declare a state of emergency over the disproportionate number of AIDS cases in the African American community. African Americans make up 15% of Alameda County, yet account for 57% of the people diagnosed with AIDS since 1980. Although HIV infections are spreading at alarming rates, silence and taboo surround HIV and AIDS within communities of color. Black and Latino youth were recruited as "town criers" on the AIDS epidemic in Alameda County, and employed the photovoice methodology to raise the prominence of this issue with the media (May, 2001).

*Flint Photovoice.* Forty-one youth and adults were recruited to document community assets and concerns, critically discuss their images, and reach policy makers. At the suggestion of grassroots community leaders, policy makers were included among those participants asked to take photographs. In accordance with established photovoice methodology, another group of policy makers and community leaders was additionally recruited to provide political will and support for implementing photovoice participants' policy and program recommendations. Flint Photovoice enabled youth to express their concerns about neighborhood violence to local policy makers, and was instrumental in acquiring funding for area violence prevention (Wang, Morrel-Samuels, Hutchison, Bell, & Pestronk, 2004).

*Youth Empowerment Strategies!* This project in Oakland, California provided 90 fifth graders with an opportunity to practice approaches in which they became actively and socially engaged in their communities. In one of the approaches, students used photovoice to document key issues in their school, their neighborhood, and their larger community. Discussions, co-facilitated by University of California at Berkeley graduate students and local high school students, enabled groups of children to focus upon issues to be promoted or remedied in their communities, leading to each group's design and implementation of a social action project. YES! Group social action projects have included several petition drives, a playground clean-up, and the formation of a first aid "Kidpatrol" at recess (Wilson, Minkler, Dasho, Carrillo, Wallerstein, & Garcia, 2006).

*Picture Me Tobacco Free©: A Youth Photovoice Action Project.* In North Carolina, this component of the Tobacco.Reality.Unfiltered campaign, supported through state tobacco settlement funds, enabled cadres of youth from participating African American Baptist churches to document the influence of tobacco within their lives and communities. Each trained Picture Me Tobacco Free© youth team sought to sponsor a photovoice exhibit at their local church and to hold an additional exhibit in a public space (Strack, Davis, Lovelace, & Holmes, 2004).

*Baltimore Youth Photovoice.* Fourteen youth involved in an after-school teen center located in the heart of a multi-ethnic community in Baltimore, Maryland participated in this photovoice project. Four exhibits showcased the work of participants, ages 11 to 17. They attended elementary, middle, and high schools, and sought to inform policy makers about issues that matter to youth living in inner cities. Strack, Magill, and McDonagh (2003) reported that parent participation in this project appeared to strengthen parent-child relationships.

*Teen Photovoice: An Educational Empowerment Program for Los Angeles Area Adolescent High School Students.* Fourteen adolescents serving on a Youth Council for the UCLA/RAND Center for Adolescent Health Promotion used digital cameras to document community influences on adolescent health behaviors. Four core themes emerged from the images taken by youth participants: food and the environment, stress and school, healthy and unhealthy relationships, and garbage in their community. Participants are now developing media products, such as posters, a video documentary, and public service announcements, in partnership with a local television station (Necheles, Wells, Hawes-Dawson, Chung, Travis, & Schuster, 2004).

*Photovoice for Tobacco, Drug and Alcohol Prevention Among Adolescents in South Africa.* Twenty-four young people in three racially diverse high schools photographed two themes: what is important in their lives, and who is important in their lives. Their work has helped to form the basis for creating youth-produced curricula on tobacco, drug, and alcohol prevention in collaboration with the Ministry of Health (Strecher, Strecher, Swart, Resnicow, & Reddy, 2004).

*Young Aboriginal People's View of Sexual Health in Western Australia.* Aboriginal youth took photographs to "show what young people (in the community) think about HIV," created narratives, and selected images for an exhibition. They identified risk behaviors, including fighting, illicit drug use, alcohol, and aspects of sexual behavior as primary HIV/AIDS risk factors. Project organizers have noted that within local public health governmental institutions, this project increased adult collaborators' respect for young people and a greater appreciation of how youth can contribute effectively to the design of health promotion strategies (Larson, Mitchell, & Gilles, 2001).

## DISCUSSION

Photovoice incorporates the community change principles identified by Checkoway (1990) of citizen participation, social action, and public advocacy, and is well-suited to youth participation. Drawing upon, and adapting, the work of Israel and colleagues on participatory action research (Israel et al., 1995), I note that specific characteristics of youth photovoice projects include: (1) the involvement of young people in all aspects of the research; (2) a co-learning process in which youth, policy makers, and researchers contribute to and learn from one another's expertise; (3) a reflective process that involves education for critical consciousness; (4) an enabling process; and (5) a balance among the goals of research, action, and evaluation. In the inter-generational Flint Photovoice in which youth, adults, and policy makers all took photographs, the youth were observed as taking to the process more easily than the policy makers, one of whom commented, "Most of us are quite good at what we do. Here we are out of our element." Facilitators observed that the use of cameras helped to even the otherwise unequal playing field with regard to participants' potential contributions (Wang, 2000).

Several youth photovoice projects noted above were "open-ended," or designed so that participants broadly photographed community issues of greatest concern to them (Photovoice Youth Empowerment Program; Flint Photovoice; Youth Empowerment Strategies!; Baltimore Youth Photovoice; Teen Photovoice). For other projects, participants were given specific themes or suggested parameters upon which to focus (Youth Violence Prevention Photovoice; Town Criers Photovoice; Picture Me Tobacco Free; Photovoice for Tobacco, Drug and Alcohol Prevention Among Adolescents in South Africa; Young Aboriginal People's View of Sexual Health in Western Australia). The former strategy facilitates youth participation in an overall community assessment; the latter approach may be used when funding or program requirements dictate a specific area focus.

The photovoice methodology facilitates youth-adult partnerships in which each group may gain insights into each others' worlds from which they are ordinarily insulated. Youth benefit from participating in the design and critique of policies and programs that directly affect their lives. Adults benefit by recognizing the skills and expertise of young people in contributing to the creation of policies and programs that are relevant and appropriate in content characteristics ranging from youth vernacular to needs and implementation.

For at least one project, youth voices were found to be effective for garnering media attention. In the San Francisco Bay area, Town Criers Photovoice generated a total of 9 television stories, three print media stories, and one radio story in the San Francisco Bay area, including a Sunday full front-page story in San Francisco's major daily (May, 2001).

Despite the potential appeal of using a camera, facilitators working with youth in a range of photovoice projects have noted challenges. Some facilitators found that youth participants may require significant encouragement in completing project activities (Stevenson, 2002; Strack, Magill, & McDonagh, 2003). Strack, Magill, and McDonagh (2003) reported that personal and family crises related to health, housing, and substance use, and stressors and competing demands, created challenges to participation for young people as well as their parents (2006). Wilson, Minkler, Dasho, Carrillo, Wallerstein, and Garcia (2006) have noted that it was important for facilitators working with a fifth grade age cohort to build in opportunities for the children's physical movement and play.

Youth participation in photovoice projects raises special ethical considerations. Wang and Redwood-Jones (2001) specify for the photovoice methodology the use of three types of written consent forms, summarized below, and in Table 2.

- Consent 1–youth photographers' signed consent to participate in project; this consent details his or her rights and responsibilities; parent or guardian must give signed consent if the young person is a minor.
- Consent 2–subjects' consent to be photographed; this consent is a signature obtained by the youth photographer and granted by any subjects *prior* to having their photograph taken.
- Consent 3–youth photographers give signed permission for pictures to be published or disseminated to promote the project's goals; this consent is usually given after all the photographs have been developed and discussed, and youth photographers have collectively identified images they wish to disseminate (Wang & Redwood-Jones, 2001).

The vulnerability of youth participants, such as through their potential tendency to downplay risks or adverse consequences of incriminating photographs, makes it essential that a parent or guardian consent signature be obtained if the youth photographer is a minor. Equally important, project facilitators are responsible for ensuring that youth participants understand that their immediate safety is paramount, and for taking every precaution possible to help minimize risks. The article "Photovoice Ethics" is critical reading for ethically implementing a

TABLE 2. Three Kinds of Consent Used in Each Photovoice Project

| Type of consent | Who obtains this type of consent? | Who gives or denies this type of consent? | When is this consent obtained? |
|---|---|---|---|
| Youth photographer's consent to participate in project; this consent details the youth photographer's rights and responsibilities | Project leader or facilitator | Youth photographer<br>If youth photographer is a minor, a parent or guardian must also provide signed consent | First workshop with youth photographers |
| Individual's consent to be photographed | Each youth photographer who photographs a human being | Each person photographed who is identifiable<br>If person photographed is a minor, a parent or guardian must also provide signed consent | *Before* an individual has his/her photograph taken |
| Youth photographer's consent to allow specific images to be published and/or disseminated | Project leader or facilitator | Participant-photographer | After all the photographs have been developed and discussed |

photovoice project involving any age group (Wang & Redwood-Jones, 2001).

Youth involvement in photovoice harnesses the desire of young people to exercise autonomy and express creativity while documenting their lives. Photovoice enables young people–including those who may be underrepresented, labeled, or stigmatized, and those of "different communities and subcommunities" (Gutiérrez, 1997)–to advocate their concerns using their language and experiences. In drawing upon youth expertise, these photovoice projects concurrently promote meaningful inter-generational partnerships and infuse youth perspectives into the process of policy and program design.

Spanning all of childhood through maturity, the term "youth" includes young people with a wide range of cognitive development, socioeconomic status, ethnicity, physical ability, sexual orientation, geography, life opportunities, and many other characteristics. Much remains to be explored regarding important differences in the way that photovoice can be most effectively adapted and used by such a diversity of young individuals. In addition, because of the lightening speed in which a person of any age can become an "unwilling and embarrassed Web celebrity" (Feuer & George, 2005), the moral and privacy rights of young people and the use of their images on the Internet–not only as photovoice photographers but also as subjects–needs further scrutiny. Finally, the dilemma associated with the challenges of evaluating the relationship between youth photovoice participation and beneficial longitudinal outcomes demands more comprehensive study. Future youth and intergenerational photovoice projects will ideally incorporate youth culture, energy, and ideas into policy and program development to build a more healthful and democratic society.

## REFERENCES

Checkoway, B. (1990). Six strategies of community change. *Community Development Journal*, 5-34.

Cottrell, B.W. (2005). Photovoice youth empowerment program. Public Health Database Results. Retrieved May 2, 2005, from the National Association of City and County Health Officials Web site: http://archive.naccho.org/modelPractices/Result.asp?PracticeID=98

Feuer, A., & George, J. (2005, February 26). Internet fame is cruel mistress for a dancer of the Numa Numa [Electronic version]. *New York Times*.

Gutiérrez, L. (1997). Multicultural community organizing. In E. Gambrill & M. Reisch (Eds.), *Social work practice in the 21st century*. Pine Forge Press.

Israel, B.A., Cummings, K.M., Dignan, M.B., Heaney, C.A., Perales, D.P., Simons-Morton, B.G., & Zimmerman, M.A. (1995). Evaluation of health education programs: Current assessment and future directions. *Health Education Quarterly, 22*, 364-389.

Killion, C.M., & Wang, C.C. (2000). Linking African American mothers across life stage and station through photovoice. *Journal of Health Care for the Poor and Underserved, 11* (3), 310-325.

Larson, A., Mitchell, E., & Gilles, M. (2001). Looking, listening, and learning about young aboriginal people's view of sexual health in Carnarvon, Western Australia: A photovoice project. Summary Report. Combined Universities Center for Rural Health. Geraldton, Western Australia.

May, M. (2001, November 25). Sounding the alarm: East Bay's teenage 'Town Criers' use cameras to bring new focus to AIDS. *San Francisco Chronicle*, p. A1.

Morrel-Samuels, S., Wang C.C., Bell, L., & Monk, C. (2005). Youth against violence: A community-based photovoice project: Summary Report. University of Michigan School of Public Health. Ann Arbor, Michigan.

Necheles, J.W., Welles, K., Hawes-Dawson, J., Chung, E., Travis, R., & Schuster, M.A. (2004). Teen photovoice: An educational empowerment program for Los Angeles area adolescent high school students. American Public Health Association Annual Meeting, Washington, DC.

Stevenson, K.Y. (2002). Town criers' photovoice project. Summary Report for The California Wellness Foundation and The Public Health Institute. Oakland, California.

Strack, R.W., Davis, T., Lovelace, K.A., & Holmes, A.P. (2004). Picture me tobacco free©: A youth photovoice action project. American Public Health Association Annual Meeting, Washington, DC.

Strack, R.W., Magill, C., & McDonagh, K. (2003). Engaging youth through photovoice. *Health Promotion Practice, 5*(1), 49-58.

Strecher, V.J., Strecher, R.H., Swart, D., Resnicow, K., & Reddy, P. (2004). Photovoice for tobacco, drug, and alcohol prevention among adolescents in South Africa. Paper presented at the Conference on Qualitative Research, University of Michigan.

Tom-Quinn, A. (2002) Understanding the new. Youth against violence photovoice. Summary Report. Ann Arbor, Michigan.

Wang, C., Burris, M., & Xiang, Y.P. (1996). Chinese village women as visual anthropologists: A participatory approach to reaching policymakers. *Social Science and Medicine, 42*, 1391-1400.

Wang, C., Yuan, Y.L., & Feng, M.L. (1996). Photovoice as a tool for participatory evaluation: The community's view of process and impact. *Journal of Contemporary Health, 4*, 47-49.

Wang, C.C. (1999). Photovoice: A participatory action research strategy applied to women's health. *Journal of Women's Health, 8*(2), 185-19.

Wang, C.C. (Ed.). (2000). *Strength to be: Community visions and voices.* University of Michigan, Ann Arbor.

Wang, C.C. (2003). Using photovoice as a participatory assessment and issue selection tool: A case study with the homeless in Ann Arbor. In M. Minkler & N. Wallerstein

(Eds.), *Community-based participatory research for health*. San Francisco: Jossey-Bass.

Wang, C.C., & Burris, M. (1997). Photovoice: Concept, methodology, and use for participatory needs assessment. *Health Education and Behavior, 24*(3), 369-387.

Wang, C.C., Cash, J., & Powers, L.S. (2000). Who knows the streets as well as the homeless?: Promoting personal and community action through photovoice. *Health Promotion Practice, 1*(1), 81-89.

Wang, C.C., Morrel-Samuels, S., Hutchison, P., Bell, L., & Pestronk, R.M. (2004). Flint photovoice: Community-building among youth, adults, and policy makers. *American Journal of Public Health, 94*(6), 911-913.

Wang, C.C, & Pies, C.A. (2004). Family, maternal, and child health through photovoice. *Maternal and Child Health Journal, 8*(2), 95-102.

Wang, C.C., & Redwood-Jones, Y. (1997). Photovoice ethics. *Health Education and Behavior, 24*(3), 369-387.

Wang, C.C, Wu, K.Y., Zhan, W.T., & Carovano, K. (1998). Photovoice as a participatory health promotion strategy. *Health Promotion International, 13*(1), 75-86.

Wilson, N., Minkler, M., Dasho, S., Carrillo, R., Wallerstein, N., & Garcia, D. (2006). Training students as partners in community based participatory prevention research: The Youth Empowerment Strategies (YES!) project. *Journal of Community Practice, 14* (1/2), 199-216.

# Participatory Action Research with Youth in Bosnia and Herzegovina

Reima Ana Maglajlić, MASW
Jennifer Tiffany, RN, MRP, PhD

**SUMMARY.** Sparked by a global UNICEF initiative, Bosnia and Herzegovina launched a participatory action research process in which 75 young people in three towns explored local understandings, needs, and actions about HIV/AIDS, drug use, human rights, and other issues. This article chronicles the research process, the action recommendations generated by young people, and the current status of the project. It reflects on the commitments and efforts which are required when large, adult-directed organizations decide to promote youth participation, and

Reima Ana Maglajlić is Freelance Consultant, Bolnika 32/IV, Flat 22, 71 000 Sarajevo, Bosnia and Herzegovina (E-mail: rea@bih.net.ba). Jennifer Tiffany is Director, HIV/AIDS Education Project, Cornell University, FLDC, Beebe Hall, Ithaca, NY 14853 USA (E-mail: jst5@cornell.edu).

The authors would like to acknowledge the contributions of the RTK BiH team 2003 (listed alphabetically): Alidzanovic, L., Buncic, R., Delibasic, B., Dragic, S., Hrkalovic, Dz., Hukic, N., Jelacic, E., Kukolj, S., Matovic, D., Mirascic, E., Mujanovic, L., Saric, S., Trninic, J., Ustovic, K., Zulic, N. and Zarchin, J.

All translations are original and were done by the first author.

The authors would also like to thank Bridgit Elizabeth Burns, Cornell University class of 2006, for her editorial assistance, and Adenike Olaode, Cornell University class of 2003, for her assistance with developing focus group questions.

[Haworth co-indexing entry note]: "Participatory Action Research with Youth in Bosnia and Herzegovina." Maglajlić, Reima Ana, and Jennifer Tiffany. Co-published simultaneously in *Journal of Community Practice* (The Haworth Press, Inc.) Vol. 14, No. 1/2, 2006, pp. 163-181; and: *Youth Participation and Community Change* (ed: Barry N. Checkoway, and Lorraine M. Gutiérrez) The Haworth Press, Inc., 2006, pp. 163-181. Single or multiple copies of this article are available for a fee from The Haworth Document Delivery Service [1-800-HAWORTH, 9:00 a.m. - 5:00 p.m. (EST). E-mail address: docdelivery@haworthpress.com].

on the institutional changes necessary to support sustained youth participation that benefits ordinary youth rather than a selected few.    *[Article
copies available for a fee from The Haworth Document Delivery Service:
1-800-HAWORTH. E-mail address: <docdelivery@haworthpress.com> Website: <http://
www.HaworthPress.com> © 2006 by The Haworth Press, Inc. All rights reserved.]*

**KEYWORDS.** Participatory action research, HIV/AIDS, adolescents,
youth

## INTRODUCTION

What's the best way to support young people to take part in activities
and processes that concern their lives? What kind of commitment and
effort does it take when an organization decides to promote and support:

- Youth Participation?
- Participatory Action Research?

How can this be done effectively in a large, complex organization? This
article explores these questions in the context of our experiences working
with the UNICEF "What every adolescent has a right to know" (RTK) initiative implemented in Bosnia and Herzegovina during 2003-2004
(UNICEF, 2003). RTK focuses on providing young people with basic information that they need to know in order to protect their health.

In April 2003, as part of the RTK initiative, the UNICEF Office in
Bosnia and Herzegovina (BiH) initiated a Participatory Action Research
(PAR) process in order to develop a communication strategy for the prevention of HIV/AIDS among adolescents in BiH. BiH is the 16th country
to be involved in the worldwide initiative. The aims of the initiative are:

- To develop a communication strategy for the prevention of
  HIV/AIDS among young people in each country where it was initiated, and
- To increase the capacity of young people to become involved in
  developing knowledge and practices that support their well-being.

The RTK initiative stipulated the use of PAR tools as a means of facilitating meaningful involvement by young people. The overall focus
of the research was determined by UNICEF headquarters, the research

was launched simultaneously in multiple countries as a result of the global initiative, and young people in all of the RTK countries took on the responsibility of carrying the research forward. This context shaped the dynamics of the PAR. The process that unfolded in BiH reflects the many constraints and opportunities created when a global adult-directed institution sparks local, youth-centered action research (Goto et al., 2003). This article reflects on the experience of conducting the PAR during 2003, reviews the findings and recommended actions generated, and describes current activities and follow-through. We hope it can contribute to improving the ways in which adults and youth, particularly in projects sponsored by large donor organizations, can cooperate to create positive social change.

## BACKGROUND

Bosnia and Herzegovina (total population ~ 3.8 million) is located in Southeastern Europe, and was part of the former Yugoslavia. The country is still in transition after the war (1992-1996), during which between 258,000-269,000 BiH inhabitants died or went missing (129,900 Bosniaks, 72,350 Serbs, 31,060 Croats and 13,500 people of other ethnicities, comprising approximately 5.9% of the pre-war population–UNHCR, 1995a, 1998). Approximately 50% of the 1991 population changed their place of residence during the conflict; in 1995, 1,282,600 were displaced and there were 1.2 million refugees (UNHCR, 1995a, 1995b). By 1998, 816,000 persons were still displaced and 712,575 had moved abroad permanently (UNHCR, 1998). After the 1995 Dayton Peace Accords, BiH was split into two political entities, the Federation of Bosnia and Herzegovina and the Republic of Srpska; the Federation of Bosnia and Herzegovina was further split into 10 Cantons each functioning as a small state.

A full discussion of the complexity of the conditions in and transitions facing BiH is beyond the scope of this article. However, in such a context, working to support and build the capacity of young people to create policies and practices that affect their lives is a moral, practical, and ethical imperative.

RTK focuses on HIV/AIDS prevention. HIV/AIDS is an emerging issue in BiH, where there is little information about the level of HIV infection and prevalent modes of transmission (UNICEF and IOM-OIM, 2002). According to official 2004 statistics, there were 56 persons with AIDS, and 28 other HIV positive persons in BiH. Some HIV positive persons from BiH are being treated abroad, mainly in Western Europe. Women who work in the sex trade face particular risk of HIV transmission. The availability and low price of narcotics like heroin also contribute to the risk of an expanding epidemic.

Existing educational programs promoting HIV prevention in BiH are mainly implemented through joint initiatives of international institutions like UNAIDS, UNICEF, and WHO and local non-governmental organizations. These programs, although aimed at supporting young people, are mainly developed and directed by adults. They often fail to address the needs and interests of young people and lack opportunities for active and meaningful adolescent participation. Young people involved in the RTK project stated that, in most HIV prevention projects, *"young people are solely a target group for second hand information, which is presented in a stereotypical and dull way (i.e., by adults holding lectures or in brochures on different topics that were developed by adults), rather than active partners for programme implementation"* (Maglajlić and RTK PAR BiH Team, 2004). Other issues include lack of donor interest in prevention programs; lack of support by governmental organizations and the media; and a tendency to focus on HIV/AIDS as an isolated issue, neglecting other important problems young people face (Maglajlić and RTK PAR BiH Team, 2004).

## RTK/BOSNIA-HERZEGOVINA

Young people involved in the RTK project in BiH identified two elements that make this initiative significantly different from other HIV/AIDS prevention programs carried out in BiH to date:

1. RTK enables young people to be meaningfully involved in the exploration of relevant issues and in the development and implementation of a country-wide prevention strategy. All of the initiatives carried out prior to this project were designed and conducted primarily by older people, emphasizing the value of professional views and experiences. Adolescents were involved in tokenistic ways, such as participation in a limited number of predefined activities.
2. RTK is based on a holistic and developmental approach to HIV/AIDS issues. In the RTK initiative, the research and action may focus on any of the 10 topics that were proposed by UNICEF

as related to HIV/AIDS–HIV/AIDS itself, sexually transmitted infections (STIs), teenage pregnancy prevention, sexuality, male and female adolescent physical development, gender issues, violence, substance misuse, human rights, and livelihoods. This approach is based on the theory that any activity that aims to provide young people with knowledge regarding these issues is also working towards the prevention of HIV/AIDS. For example, efforts that help prevent breaches of adolescents' human rights can contribute to HIV/AIDS prevention. The young people conducting the research chose to focus their studies on topics about which the youth in their towns had the least knowledge and on issues where there appeared to be the greatest need.

## THE PAR PROCESS

### Division of Responsibilities

The first part of the RTK PAR in Bosnia and Herzegovina was carried out between May and December 2003 by teams of young people in three towns (Tuzla, Banja Luka, and Sarajevo; see Figure 1) supported by a head researcher (Rea Maglajlić). UNICEF/BiH provided funding and overall supervision for the project. A "peer debriefer" from Cornell University (Jennifer Tiffany) used email to communicate with the head researcher and offered consultation on evaluating and sustaining the effort.

FIGURE 1. Structure of RTK PAR BiH

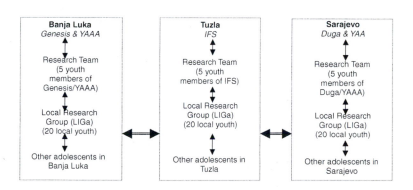

*Research Teams.* In each of the three sites, the partner organizations (Youth Action Against AIDS and Genesis from Banja Luka, Duga and Youth Against AIDS from Sarajevo, and International Forum of Solidarity from Tuzla) nominated a team of five local young people from within their membership to serve as the Research Team. The Research Team members were paid part-time for their work. They facilitated the PAR process with the members of the Local Research Group, LIGa (see below). Facilitation tasks were separated into different roles, such as facilitating activities during meetings, keeping record (audio and written) and/or playing "the devil's advocate" to make sure that difficult issues were aired. The Team members took turns in these roles, according to a joint agreement and interest. Team members also wrote reports and had the overall responsibility of making sure the work stayed focused on project objectives.

*Local Research Groups (LIGa).* During May 2003, each of the Research Teams established a Local Research Group (*lokalna istrazivaćka grupa* or LIGa in Bosnian). Each LIGa involved 15-20 young people from the participating town who were interested in the research topic(s) and had time to take part in the project. The average age of LIGa members was 17, with a range from 13-19. At the time of the study, all of the LIGa members were still in school. Fifty to seventy percent of co-researchers in each town were female. Each research Team developed their own strategy about who would be invited to join the LIGa; since they aimed to establish diverse and representative groups, suggestions included young people who misused substances, youth who had lost parents in the war, youth involved in sports and athletics, youth from different religious groups, and LGBTQ youth. Each group was formed drawing on personal contacts of Team members. Even though the LIGas reflected the desired diversity, members did not join to serve as representatives of a particular demographic sub-set but as youth from their towns, interested in the aims of the project. LIGa members noted the following reasons for joining:

- doing something useful for their communities
  *Since we try to solve problems in our town.* (members of the LIGa in Tuzla)
- it's an opportunity to learn something new and become more confident
  *It is a kind of additional education.* (members of the LIGa in Banja Luka)

*To become more confident and develop work habits.* (members of the LIGa in Sarajevo)
- to meet new friends and spend time with them
- to earn money.

Each of the LIGa members received a small payment (100 Bosnian Konvertible Marks or $62 US; the average monthly income in BiH is approximately 450KM, or $280 US.)

The LIGa members, together with the Research Team, decided what to research, how to research it, with whom and when. They conducted the research and other activities with other adolescents in their town, made sense of the data, and worked with the Research Team to develop the proposal for a prevention strategy.

During a focus group discussion about their participation held during late 2003, LIGa members recognized their central role in carrying out the work and that they had done a good job, primarily since they co-operated with each other.

> *We developed trust in each other, came up with ideas for our work, we were all great.* (members of the Sarajevo LIGa)

> *We conducted the research, organized and implemented the activities, distributed information to other adolescents, etc.* (members of the Tuzla LIGa)

> *We did the research, we spent time with our peers, we did the toughest part of the work. We exchanged experiences and information and made it all so good and original.* (members of the Banja Luka LIGa)

*Head Researcher.* The head researcher's role was to build the capacity of the Research Team members to conduct the PAR process with their peers and to supervise their work. The role was perceived as that of someone who supports and monitors the work, and acts as a link between the LIGa members, Research Teams and UNICEF.

> *She's a connection between the sharing group and UNICEF, someone who supports our ideas and monitors our work, she's great.* (members of the Sarajevo LIGa)

UNICEF. UNICEF's role was recognized as crucial in terms of initiating and funding the work. The organization was also seen as a source of support, despite some difficulties such as delays in payments and distribution of materials. In fact, one of the Sarajevo meetings was postponed due to a strike by the young people because of a delay in payment. Such delays were a regular occurrence for all three BiH sites and were also reported as an issue in other RTK projects (Goto et al., 2003). However, the central role of UNICEF as an initiator of this type of work, unique for the BiH context, was recognized.

> *They took care of the funding. If they weren't here, this project wouldn't take place. They were the support–a foreign element that gave our ideas an opportunity to develop. They had really strong motivation to show the world that BiH is doing something and that we are capable and knowledgeable to do it. They believed in us.* (The Banja Luka LIGa)

The RTK process in BiH was complex, and substantial attention was paid to the quality of collaboration among young people and adults involved in the project, as well as to the quality of the PAR study itself. Following specific suggestions by Heron (1996), this PAR process was designed so that participants would move through several cycles of reflection and action and learn to balance reflection and action. This was achieved by conducting small scale research and practice activities, critiquing them as a group, and then developing another round of research and activities drawing upon what had been learned. The participants also produced a practical nation-wide communication strategy and proposed that they be involved in its implementation in 2004.

### Meetings

Each Team and the LIGa members met nine times during a six-month period (June-December 2003). Meetings were scheduled at times that didn't conflict with school or other responsibilities of the LIGa or Team members. On average, extended meetings took place every 2-3 weeks.

The head researcher and Research Team members met before and after each of the LIGa meetings. At the "pre-meeting," the Team members practiced their duties for the LIGa meetings and made any necessary amendments to the planned agenda. During the "post meeting," they reflected on the LIGa meeting (what went well, what didn't go so well, what could be done to improve the next meeting), drafted an agenda for the following meeting, and defined the roles Team members would play in facilitating it. The head researcher was present at the majority of the meetings, mainly as an observer. LIGa members described the work as a supportive, collaborative process. In the focus group that was organized as part of the project's evaluation, the LIGa members said they saw the Team members as colleagues who coordinated the work, as more active LIGa members, rather than as hierarchically above the LIGa; the head researcher was recognized for her ability to facilitate communications, provide technical support, and, as someone in her thirties, to bridge the gap between adults and young people.

> *They gave us instructions on how to conduct research. They educated us, gathered our information and summarized it for us. They were good and strong support and they coordinated our work.* (Members of the Banja Luka LIGa)

> *She listens and doesn't speak; then she asks a good question for discussion. She's not someone who opposes us; she's like a member of the LIGa. She does her job well and has a good car. She controls the quality of our work, and makes sure we do everything on time. She was good.* (Members of the Banja Luka LIGa)

The 15 Research Team members from all three towns had a "half-way" meeting in early August 2003 to exchange experiences and plan the PAR process for the rest of the year. In November 2003, all of the 75 co-researchers met in Sarajevo to share their findings to date with various stakeholders (UNICEF BiH representatives, representatives of relevant governmental and non-governmental organizations, the media, etc.) and to jointly plan future project activities.

## Research Questions, Methods, and Findings

The research topics, methods, and questions used in all three towns are summarized in Figure 2.

Each town took developed a unique approach to the research. For example, in Tuzla the LIGa and Team members conducted a qualitative survey among parents and raised funds independently to hold a two-day basketball tournament for young people entitled "No drugs, no alcohol, just play basketball." LIGa members conducted the activity because they had identified boredom and a lack of free time activities as one of the main reasons for high rates of substance misuse among their peers.

FIGURE 2. Research Topics, Questions, and Methods

**Research topics selected:**

Banja Luka - Sexually transmitted infections and human rights
Sarajevo - Sexually transmitted infections and HIV/AIDS
Tuzla - Substance misuse

**Research questions:**

What do adolescents know about the research topic? What don't they know?

What are the risk behaviors associated with the topic? Why do adolescents expose themselves to these risks, despite the knowledge they have about the topic?

How do adolescents want to receive further information about this topic? By whom? Where? When (how often)? Why?

**Research methods:**

Qualitative and quantitative surveys
*(The LIGa and Team members devised the questionnaires, determined the sample, prepared and carried out the fieldwork, analyzed the results and, through group discussion, utilized them to prepare the communication strategy.)*

PAR tools adapted from Gregoire et al. (2003) and Tiffany et al. (1993)

Group discussions

Activities with other adolescents

Seventy-two couples took part in the tournament, and many youth attended the event as spectators. During breaks between games, there were performances by young dancers, and each night young DJs organized a party. Throughout the day, LIGa members distributed brochures on substance misuse, HIV/AIDS prevention, and condoms. They also used this opportunity to collect some information through "comment walls," where young people shared their opinions on different topics like safer sex and ways to overcome boredom.

The PAR process explored factual knowledge, factors underlying factual knowledge, and actual behaviors (see Figure 2). Adolescents generally had some basic knowledge of about the issues being researched. For example, they knew that they can get sexually transmitted infections (STIs) through unprotected sexual intercourse. However, they lacked detailed knowledge about treatment and prevention, such as:

- different types of STIs,
- symptoms for different STIs,

- how STIs can be cured, and
- which sexual activities put you at most risk to get a STI.

Adolescents had more detailed knowledge of substance misuse issues than of other explored topics. Parents reported that they were sufficiently informed about the research issues, but adolescents didn't agree. Adolescents said that parents often ignore what is happening in their children's lives until a crisis occurs.

Through the PAR activities, young people identified several different factors that contributed to risky behaviors. The Team summarized their findings as follows:

- *You can't have a life without any risks*
  Adolescents are curious and don't think about the consequences of their behaviors. They often think *"it can't happen to me."* Taking part in risky behaviors attracts peer attention and sometimes increases the social standing of the young person.
- *Socio-economic context*
- The wide availability of addictive substances fosters substance misuse.
- The tenuous socio-economic situation in the country creates intense stress, economic insecurity, and incentives for participating in commercial sex work or for using narcotics: *"If you don't have enough money, you can prostitute yourself to earn it. Or a friend of your's can offer you drugs. It's a comfort thing."* (members of the Sarajevo LIGa)
- *Boredom*
  Young people lack opportunities to earn money due to the socio-economic situation, and also need better free time activities. They mainly spend time listening to music, watching TV or hanging out with their friends. They have nothing interesting to do in their spare time.
- *Low self-esteem*
  "Low self-esteem" was one of the most commonly identified reasons for risky behavior. Young people believed it was caused by the following factors:
- Adolescents don't see any future for themselves in BiH: *"We live in the past, constantly looking back on what happened to us, instead of planning our future. We don't see it, at least not here."*
- Problems in the education system: Teachers often lack professionalism and use class time to vent their personal problems.

- Pressures on all society members due to the poor socio-economic situation in BiH
- Bad experiences with their parents
- Other factors like socio-economic pressures combine with low self-esteem to create the following attitude *"It can't happen to me, but if it does, it doesn't matter since my life is irrelevant anyway and is leading nowhere."* The low self-esteem among young women makes them more likely to consent to unprotected sex in fear of losing a partner or to sexual intercourse with significantly older men.

- *Educational system policies and problems*

- Sex and condom use are mentioned for the first time in the second year of high-school and there is little discussion of such issues in the school context. Teachers or other lecturers often use old-fashioned lecture-type presentations, without any attempts for active student involvement or dialogue. Further, schools may not be perceived as a credible source of information because of widespread corruption in the education system. The researchers found that, in some schools, you can buy a good grade for a certain amount of money.

- *Patriarchal society*

- We live in a patriarchal society that strictly defines the roles of young women and men. These roles are learned in the family and lead to young women's vulnerability to risky behaviors and violence.

- *Traditional values*

- There are many contradictions between traditional values and the reality of young people's lives. For example, the norm that they are not to enter into sexual relationships prior to marriage is widely known but rarely practiced. Adolescents are ideally expected to behave as children and are not given the liberty to make independent decisions. For example, if a young woman visits a gynecologist, she is considered to be irresponsible (since she's engaging in sexual intercourse), rather than responsible since she is taking care of her health. Also, if an adolescent is seen buying condoms at the local shop, the shopkeeper is likely to tell his/her parents about the young person's "shameful behavior." Young people fear community reactions if they are to tell anyone that they have an STI or HIV/AIDS. They are afraid of stigma and isolation.

The PAR also explored factors that support healthy behavior changes. One major positive influence identified was joining forces with peers–joint support and learning helps keep young people healthy. Our experiences during the RTK PAR are one example of such cooperation.

### Assessing the Group Process

The monitoring and evaluation exercises conducted during December 2003 indicated that young people appreciated the following aspects of participating in RTK:

- team and group work, particularly the honesty and the openness of group members
- *Everyone who is here talks really openly and without fear, hoping that we will help other adolescents through our work.* (Banja Luka LIGa member)
- expressing their opinions and finding them accepted
- *Every member of the group has a right to say what s/he thinks, regardless of how old s/he is.* (Tuzla LIGa member)
- the way we work–creative, active work in a relaxed atmosphere
- *I liked the way we prepared the survey and chose the questions for it.* (Sarajevo LIGa member)
- company, particularly of the opposite gender.

Many young people were positive about the relevance and potential they had as a group. This contrasts with many of the Team's findings regarding self-esteem, lack of hope for the future, and young people's sense of not feeling valued in the present. Still, some co-researchers (particularly young women) rated the importance of their individual contributions lower than the group's collective capacity.

### Proposed Actions

Based on the PAR, young people identified two main priorities for future prevention activities.

*Peer Education.* The only way for communication activities to involve the majority of the adolescent population in BiH would be to implement a nation-wide, school-based peer education program. Young people found participatory peer education to be the best way to raise awareness and inform their peers about the issues explored in RTK. They emphasized the key role of the *approach* utilized in peer education (see also Goto et al., 2003; Goto, 2004); it should be conducted through group-based, interactive workshops, which would be mandatory, but not graded. Currently, professionals (teachers, health workers) don't have an effective approach when carrying out these activities. Peer education should be implemented beginning in late elementary school and continuing through graduation from high school.

*Cooperation with the Media.* At all sites the co-researchers confirmed the significant role of the media in young people's lives and explored how media can best be utilized in a national HIV/AIDS prevention communication strategy. Specific ideas proposed by the teams included:

- Talk shows which would enable adolescents, parents, teachers and other stakeholders to explore the practical implications of the problems they face in day to day life in relation to the RTK topics (like the increased substance misuse among adolescents or breaches of adolescents' and teachers' human rights in schools) and offer possible practical solutions based on the needs and preferences of adolescents.
- TV advertisements with the following qualities:
  continuous (i.e., year long) series of ads
  cartoon or live characters who would, through a series of brief stories, promote a healthy lifestyle (this way, there would be a common thread throughout the campaign, while constantly recapturing the attention of both adolescents and their parents).
- Billboards

  A good way to promote the healthy lifestyle messages among both adolescents and their parents.

- Music

  At the final 2003 workshop, with help from the UNICEF staff, we invited music stars from BiH and the surrounding region to learn about our work–Toše Proeski (a pop star from Macedonia who serves as UNICEF's Regional RTK ambassador), Edo Maajka (a rap artist) and Zabranjeno Pušenje (a rock band). Young people presented the PAR findings to the musicians who will make songs to promote the findings to adolescents and their parents. We selected music stars who are listened to by both the young people and their parents, and who represent different music styles.

*Extending the RTK PAR Process to Younger and Rural Youth.* The PAR process conducted during 2003 was brief in duration and involved adolescents from only three towns. The young people proposed conducting a second round of PAR during 2004, involving younger youth (12-15 year olds) from rural areas. The young people involved during 2003 would take on an even stronger role in facilitating research in rural areas near their towns, with less "hands-on" support from the head researcher and increased opportunities to test and to develop their planning, facilitation, and research capabilities. Implementing the PAR process with rural youth and adults would address major gaps in knowledge about conditions facing young people in BiH.

*Crosscutting* all three of these proposals is the strong recommendation from both the Team and LIGa members for continuing the involvement of the original group at the same time as creating opportunities for additional young people to join in. This sustained involvement would allow continuing members to practice their new capabilities in different situations, and further develop their sense of capacity while also extending the capacity-building process to larger numbers of youth.

## FOLLOW-UP AND RECOMMENDATIONS

Most of the work described in this article occurred during the last eight months of 2003. The first RTK initiative ended in December 2003. Here is a brief update about 2004 follow-up project activities in BiH.

*Rural PAR.* The recommended rural PAR was conducted in communities near Banja Luka and Tuzla starting in mid-2004, facilitated by youth researchers who built upon the skills and insights they developed during 2003. Although the contract for the work was approved fairly quickly, given the size and complexity of the funding organization, the months-long delay in following through on this recommendation broke the morale and momentum of the young people involved. Some of them were able to, in part, compensate for this by initiating planning and community-based meetings even before the formal agreement with UNICEF was in place.

*Media.* Adult media consultants were hired to develop and implement media based on the PAR findings. There was no further involvement of youth from the RTK teams. The rationale was that the initial focus of the RTK PAR process was to develop broad guidelines and a research base for a national communication strategy, rather than to create and implement the strategy. Nonetheless, this marks a lost opportunity for innovative adult-youth collaboration, and for the development of an additional set of skills among young people committed to the project.

*Peer Education.* The RTK Team recommended that one way to develop a nation-wide peer education strategy, building upon the capacity of the young researchers to work in partnership with adults, would be to convene working groups of stakeholders. Using this approach, youth who had experience with the RTK PAR process would collaborate with additional youth, parents, teachers, faculty of universities that educate teachers, and other stakeholders in the design of policies and programs on the local level. Due to the devolved governmental structure in BiH, such a proposal made sense both practically and strategically. This plan was initially agreed upon by both youth and UNICEF representatives in late 2003. However, in mid-2004 UNICEF instead initiated a peer education mapping and data gathering exercise, in partnership with another youth organization, the Youth Information Agency. A few representatives from the RTK 2003 Teams are members of the Work Group but do not have a leadership or advisory role in the project.

This brings us squarely to discussion of the role of large organizations (including supranational agencies) in supporting youth participation on any level, from grassroots up. These are crucial questions, because, while youth participation is a "hot" global and national issue, the emphasis on involving young people has too often resulted in little or no benefit to the lives of ordinary youth. The insights generated in BiH can help to guide us towards interventions that have deeper and more sustained benefits for larger numbers of youth.

*Allow Enough Time.* One issue encountered in RTK BiH (and in many other initiatives) is the short duration of the project–intense involvement of young people for a few months, followed by either a termination of the effort or uncertainty as to what will happen next. Such a situation is similar to that in many non-governmental programs in BiH. On average, work in NGOs is geared towards short-term project implementation, with an average duration of about 6-12 months (ICVA, 2002). While much was accomplished between May and December 2003, a longer period of engagement would have been more constructive on several grounds: (1) Young people could have solidified their new capabilities. (2) Particularly in contexts like BiH, it is vital that young people develop a sense of security and of self-efficacy–both of which are jeopardized by brief, time-limited interventions. (3) Young people could enter into working partnerships with adults, contributing to the development of effective policies and programs as well as to other skills needed for democratic practice. (4) Community coalitions supporting continued youth engagement would have had time to emerge and to become institutionalized. We recommend that organizations commit to, at minimum, two years of sustained support.

*Create Flexibility.* There can be a clash between the flexibility demanded by doing participatory work with young people and the normal demands of large bureaucracies. Exacerbating this clash, large organizations often have vague definitions of youth participation, and little opportunity to examine what authentic youth participation demands in terms of staff, policies, and procedures. At the same time, the insights and concerns of young people may help large agencies to do a more adequate job of administering their resources. Youth in several RTK countries went on short-term strikes in response to procedural issues (inadequate reimbursement for travel expenses, delayed finalization of contracts with local NGOs) (Goto et al., 2003; Maglajlić and RTK PAR Team, 2004) that adults may have been less likely to protest.

*Define the Role and Unique Capacities of Large Organizations.* In the case of RTK, UNICEF occupied in a unique position in relation to parallel PAR efforts being conducted simultaneously among young people on many continents. To some extent, organizational roles and responsibilities were defined only as the initiative unfolded. Throughout, young people made it clear that one important role for UNICEF (or any donor organizations that sparks new initiatives in multiple sites) lies in facilitating contact among teams who are geographically and culturally distant from one another. Young people clearly stated their passion for knowing what their peers and colleagues were doing, in nearby communities and halfway across the globe. Keiko Goto, reflecting on the RTK initiative, suggests two specific roles that large and supranational organizations can play: (1) creating environments at the organizational and local levels in which participatory approaches can thrive, and (2) gathering and disseminating PAR findings (Goto, 2004). Large organizations like UNICEF can not only facilitate horizontal dissemination of findings and processes among participating sites but also can ensure that the work of young people conducting PAR informs the development of policies and programs. Intra-organizational coordination and communications can be vital to dissemination of findings, but sometimes are lacking. For example, at the same time as the RTK PAR was underway in BiH, UNICEF was coordinating the country wide policy group that steered all HIV/AIDS prevention and treatment initiatives, and yet no communication was established between the two initiatives.

*Transform Power Relationships.* Who ultimately has decision making power? The policies and procedures of organizations promoting youth participation have to promote and ensure meaningful participation *within their institutions*, not just in community-level projects. This links to the issue of program planning and the extent to which efforts are sustained over time: How will the young people be involved in the decisions made about whether a project continues? This is a messy and gray area, especially given the frequent lack of cooperation and participation among adults. Again, improving practice and understanding in the area of youth participation opens doors for more authentic engagement of people of all ages.

Organizations sometimes find it easy to empower individual youth, incorporating them into existing decision-making structures and power relationships. This type of participation may engage only a few selected, well educated, eloquent youth who speak at least one foreign language. A small number of carefully chosen youth participates in conferences and other professional activities. This mode of youth participation may create a small circle of professional youth representatives instead of enabling the shifts in power relationships, mutual cooperation and learning that are necessary for sustained and structural change. Deeper transformations would, of course, include improvement in practices around transparency and authentic participation between adults and other adults, youth and other youth, as well as between adults and youth.

In the words of the young people involved in RTK BiH:

> *The most important aspect of our work to date and, hopefully, in the next project phase is the fact that we were really and truly involved in this project. This is the aspect of the work which was the most appreciated to date, it is something that keeps us all motivated for what we do and should clearly be the most important feature of the future project activities. Both adults and young people in the project*

*had a lot to learn from each other, but the main lesson is that, given time and patience, there is very little we cannot achieve. This is an extremely important issue, particularly coming from a country such as our own, where many things happened that were out of our control, which gravely affected our lives.* (Maglajlić and the RTK BiH Team, 2004)

# REFERENCES

Goto, K. (2004). *The application of a participatory approach in health and nutrition programs: A case study of an HIV/AIDS prevention initiative among youth.* Ithaca, NY: Cornell University Doctoral Dissertation.

Goto, K. et al. (2003). *UNICEF's 'What every adolescent has a right to know': A PAR approach to HIV/AIDS prevention among youth.* Paper presented at the 2003 Action Learning, Action Research and Process Management World Congress, Pretoria, South Africa.

Gregoire, H. (Ed.), with the Cornell RTK Working Group (2003). *Participatory action research in the context of UNICEF's "What every adolescent has a right to know (RTK)" initiative–PAR toolkit.* Ithaca, NY: RTK Working Group/Cornell University HIV/AIDS Education Project.

Heron, J. (1996). *Co-operative inquiry: Research into the Human Condition.* London: Sage.

ICVA (2002). Istraćivanje nevladinog sektora u BiH (Research of the non-governmental sector in BiH), in ICVA *Pogledi na NVO sektor u BiH (A view of the NGO sector in BiH).* Sarajevo: ICVA, 22-38.

Maglajlić, R.A. and RTK PAR BiH Team (2004). Right to Know, UNICEF BiH–Developing a Communication Strategy for the Prevention of HIV/AIDS among young people through PAR. *Child Care in Practice, 10*(2), 127-139.

Tiffany, J. S., D. Tobias, A. Raqib, & J. Ziegler (1993). *Talking with kids about AIDS teaching guide.* Ithaca, NY: Cornell University Department of Human Service Studies.

UNHCR (1995a). The State of the World's Refugees.

_____. (1995b). The State of the World's Refugees Seeking Asylum.

_____. (1998) Populations of Concern to UNHCR-1997 Statistical Overview.

UNICEF (2003). *Right to Know Initiative–Global portfolio [CD-Rom].* New York, NY: UNICEF.

UNICEF and IOM-OIM (2002). *Pregled raširenosti HIV/SIDA-e u jugoistočnoj Europi: Epidemiološki podaci, ugroćene skupine, odgovori vlada I nevladinih organizacija do siječnja 2002 (Review of HIV/AIDS prevalence in SE Europe: Epidemiological data, at-risk groups and governmental and non-governmental responses until January 2002).* Sarajevo: UNICEF and IOM-OIM.

# The *Growing Up in Cities* Project:
# Global Perspectives on Children and Youth as Catalysts for Community Change

Louise Chawla, PhD
David Driskell, AICP

**SUMMARY.** The United Nations Convention on the Rights of the Child contains a set of "participation clauses" which are leading members of development agencies, municipal offices, and community organizations to incorporate children and youth into community planning. The *Growing Up in Cities* project of UNESCO provides a model for doing this, with a focus on low-income areas of special concern for urban policy-makers. The authors describe a case study of this project in Bangalore, India, explore the complexities of implementation of youth participation, and discuss the lessons learned. *[Article copies available for a fee from The Haworth Document Delivery Service: 1-800-HAWORTH. E-mail address: <docdelivery@haworthpress.com> Website: <http://www.HaworthPress.com> © 2006 by The Haworth Press, Inc. All rights reserved.]*

**KEYWORDS.** Children, youth, community development, participation, children's rights

---

Address all correspondence to: Louise Chawla, PhD, Professor, Kentucky State University, 400 East Main Street, Frankfort, KY 40601 (E-mail: louise.chawla@kysu.edu)

David Driskell, AICP, is a Lecturer in the Department of City and Regional Planning, Cornell University, Ithaca, NY.

[Haworth co-indexing entry note]: "The *Growing Up in Cities* Project: Global Perspectives on Children and Youth as Catalysts for Community Change." Chawla, Louise, and David Driskell. Co-published simultaneously in *Journal of Community Practice* (The Haworth Press, Inc.) Vol. 14. No. 1/2, 2006, pp. 183-200; and: *Youth Participation and Community Change* (ed: Barry N. Checkoway, and Lorraine M. Gutiérrez) The Haworth Press, Inc., 2006, pp. 183-200. Single or multiple copies of this article are available for a fee from The Haworth Document Delivery Service [1-800-HAWORTH, 9:00 a.m. - 5:00 p.m. (EST). E-mail address: docdelivery@haworthpress.com].

## AN INTERNATIONAL FRAMEWORK
## FOR CHILD AND YOUTH PARTICIPATION

People working on behalf of children and youth around the world are turning to a strong but flexible instrument to hold governments and institutions accountable for providing young people with the conditions they need for healthy development–including conditions that enable young people to participate in community decision-making. The Convention on the Rights of the Child, which was adopted by the United Nations General Assembly in 1989, extends basic economic, social, cultural and civil rights to everyone under the age of 18 (United Nations, 1989).[1] Most of the Convention's 54 clauses deal with familiar provisions, such as children's rights to protection from exploitation and abuse and their right to primary education. A set of "participation clauses," however, requires adults to see children and youth as partners in planning for their own well-being (Hart, 1997). (See Table 1.) This article explores an initiative to implement this right to participation in a Bangalore slum and the obstacles that limited its full realization.

As with all human rights documents, there is a difference between the Convention's high rhetoric and reality on the ground. Nevertheless, people who work with children and youth around the world believe that the Convention is contributing to a sea change in adults' perceptions of young people, and in some cases it is being used effectively as a legal mandate for the inclusion of young people in decisions that affect their lives. It is leading many decision makers to recognize young people as resourceful agents with ideas worth hearing, rather than just "incomplete adults" who are defined by what they cannot yet do.

One place where change is evident is in community development. Building on the Convention, for example, the Preamble to the United Nations Habitat Agenda states that, "Special attention needs to be paid to the participatory processes dealing with the shaping of cities, towns . and neighborhoods; this is in order to secure the living conditions of children and of youth and to make use of their insight, creativity and thoughts on the environment" (United Nations Centre for Human Settlements, 1996).[2] In response to these principles, many municipalities are currently searching for ways to integrate young people into community development processes, and one of the tools that they have found for doing this is the Growing Up in Cities project of UNESCO–the United Nations Educational, Scientific and Cultural Organization.

Conceived in 1970 by Kevin Lynch, an urban designer at MIT, the project was created to involve adolescents in evaluating their urban en-

TABLE 1. Participation Clauses of the *Convention on the Rights of the Child*

Article 12.1  States Parties shall assure to the child who is capable of forming his or her own views the right to express those views freely in all matters affecting the child, the views of the child being given due weight in accordance with the age and maturity of the child.

Article 13.1  The child shall have the right to freedom of expression; this right shall include freedom to seek, receive and impart information and ideas of all kinds, regardless of frontiers, either orally, in writing or in print, in the form of art, or through any other media of the child's choice.

Article 14.1  States Parties shall respect the right of the child to freedom of thought, conscience and religion.

Article 15.1  States Parties recognize the rights of the child to freedom of association and to freedom of peaceful assembly.

The full text of the Convention can be found at www.unicef.org/crc.htm.

vironments and making recommendations for improvements (Lynch, 1977). In response to the Convention on the Rights of the Child and the Habitat Agenda, the project was revived in 1996, and it has been steadily spreading to new sites since that time (Chawla, 2002). As this article goes to press, more than 50 sites in six continents have been documented.[3] In 1970, however, Lynch's ideas were a generation ahead of his time and city officials showed no interest in what young people had to say.

Growing Up in Cities creates model projects in areas of special concern for urban policy-makers: squatter settlements, refugee camps, areas with immigrants or ethnic minorities, and districts with high rates of poverty or alienation (Figure 1). Using a variety of methods, it involves young people in action research to document their lives and the places where they live, to explore and evaluate the issues that affect them, to prioritize their ideas for change, and to take action to make change happen (Driskell, 2002). Although some sites have engaged 8 through 18-year-olds, project sites have typically targeted ages 10 through 15. Through its program of participatory activities, Growing Up in Cities seeks to improve the conditions of young people's lives through two means: by involving young people themselves in identifying and contributing to positive changes in the programs and places that serve them, and by exposing obstacles to change. These two sides are illustrated by the story of the project's implementation in a self-built settlement in India.

FIGURE 1. The Growing Up in Cities project involves young people in action research to document their lives and the places where they live, explore and evaluate the issues that affect them, prioritize their ideas for change, and take action to make change happen. The project has been active in more than 30 sites since 1996. (Photo courtesy of Robin Moore.)

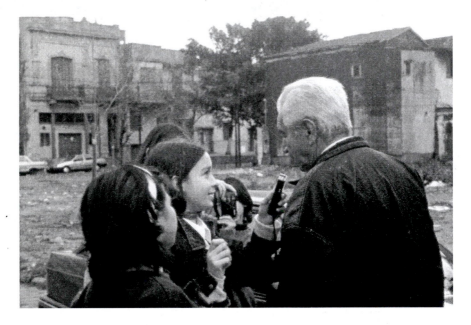

## CHILDREN'S LIVES IN "TRUTH TOWN"

The Growing Up in Cities site in India was located on the periphery of Bangalore–capital of the State of Karnataka, center of the country's booming information technology sector, and one of Asia's fastest growing cities over the past twenty years. The name of the project location, Sathyanagar, roughly translates from the original Sanskrit as 'truth' (*sathya*) 'town' (*nagar*). In retrospect, it proved to be a fitting name for a place to explore the lives and perspectives of young people and the obstacles that they and their families face in efforts to improve their situation.

Like many urban settlements in India and throughout the developing world, Sathyanagar is a place that outsiders–including many middle-class Indians–would describe as dirty, squalid, poverty-stricken and depressed (Figure 2). It is both in the classification scheme of the state bureaucracy and in the local nomenclature of its residents, a slum.

Yet this is hardly representative of the picture that emerged from young people's own stories about Sathyanagar and their lives there. Though set in the context of a comparatively poor and environmentally degraded place, their stories tell of culturally and emotionally rich, happy lives, in a community that possessed a number of advantages: some apparent, and some perhaps invisible to the eyes of its adults.

The Growing Up in Cities project in Sathyanagar worked with 38 children (18 girls and 20 boys) from the ages of 10 through 14.[4] Recruited to the project via "snowball sampling" based on initial contacts through several local NGOs and community leaders, the resulting sample of child participants were representative of a cross-section of the community's linguistic and religious groups, as well as different

FIGURE 2. The Growing Up in Cities site in Bangalore, India was a self-built settlement on the edge of the city. The project has focused primarily on very low income areas, though its methods have also been applied in middle class and mixed income communities. (Photo courtesy of David Driskell)

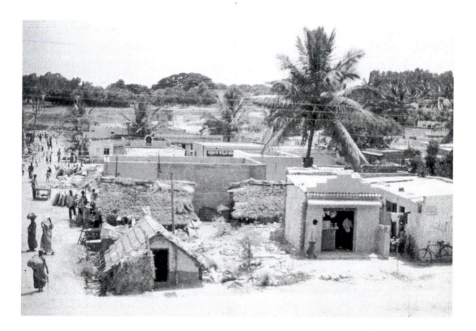

schooling and work options (a state-subsidized school, an informal school operated by a local NGO, and school drop-outs who were working full time). All of the children worked at least part-time, either in their home or nearby, and nearly all in the informal economy.

As at other project locations, the project engaged these young people in a participatory evaluation of their community using a core set of research methods. Site-based work began with a month-long period in which members of the core project team spent time informally in the settlement area, assisting in the informal school or other community activities. During this period, they were also trained in the project's more formal research methods–most notably in conducting the one-on-one interviews. The core team consisted of two young males and two young females from a local NGO, several volunteers from a local college who were earning course credit for their participation, and two project co-directors who were responsible for training and management (all of whom were part-time on the project).

Formal research activities were initiated with a drawing exercise, in which young people were asked to "make a drawing of the area where you live" (Figure 3). Members of the core project team then interviewed participants, one-on-one (Figure 4). Each interview was conducted in two sessions, requiring approximately 90 minutes, on average, to complete both sessions. In addition to discussing the drawing, the interviews included a daily time schedule (in which young people listed their activities during a recent weekday and a recent weekend day) and a social network diagram (in which they were asked to identify the family members and friends with whom they live or who they visit frequently).

Following the one-on-one interviews, a series of small group activities involved young participants in further exploration of their local area, discussions with their peers, and discussions with members of the core research team. These activities included child-led walking tours of the local area, child-taken photographs, and focus group discussions. Core team members also carried out a community survey, mapping of the site, and interviews with parents and local officials responsible for providing basic services to the community. The young participants then prepared a community exhibition of their work and findings, and helped define priorities for action (eventually resulting in construction of a new Study Center facility, as discussed later in this article).

The stories shared by Sathyanagar's young people spoke of young people living under difficult circumstances: of six and seven year-olds thrust into adult roles; of hours spent each day in household chores such as fetching potable water; of children exposed to open sewer drains in

FIGURE 3. Children are first asked to make a drawing of the area where they live. This helps illustrate their perception of the local area—what they know about it, where they go, and what they value. It also serves as the basis for the initial interview and further discussion. (Photo courtesy of David Driskell)

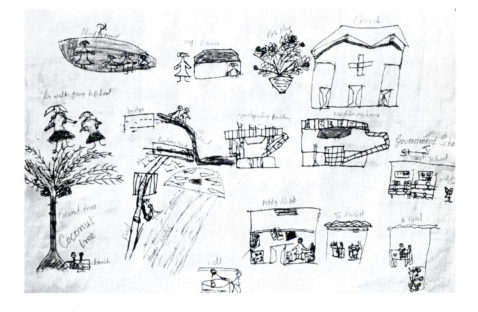

their daily play; of people's lives cut short by disease and violence; of social and political injustice. As an 11-year-old boy noted, "The gutters are dirty and there is no flow of sewage and so it stinks."

Yet, the stories from Sathyanagar also spoke of young people with an astonishing degree of resilience. In many cases, the children of Sathyanagar could be described as *confident, connected* and *happy– words seldom used to describe young people in many other Growing Up in Cities sites that enjoyed much higher relative levels of well-being* (Figure 5).

Although Sathyanagar had little financial capital, in the eyes of the project children it was rich in social and cultural capital. Despite many chores, income-generating work, and school responsibilities, the children took advantage of every spare moment to play, and they were rarely at a loss for friends or ideas. Despite their material lack of play equipment, they engaged in all manner of activities: playing tag, rolling

FIGURE 4. To understand their drawing and introduce other topics of discussion, a one-on-one interview is conducted with each child. This also helps develop participants' abilities to articulate their ideas, leading into other small group participation activities. (Photo courtesy of David Driskell)

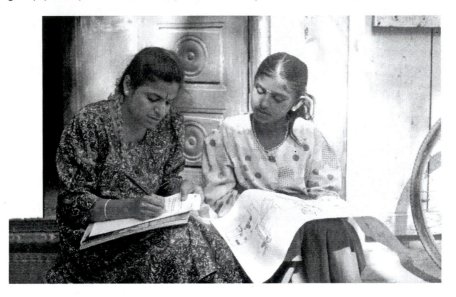

an old tire with a stick, drawing in the dirt, exploring an adjacent area, playing Gilli Dandu (a popular game played with two sticks), or even building a makeshift "temple" complete with an idol and a ceremonial *pooja* (worship service). Two large flat open spaces on the periphery of the settlement were the site for Sunday afternoon cricket tournaments, pitting teams from Sathyanagar against teams from adjacent settlements. During the several month process of conducting the participatory research activities, not a single child in Sathyanagar was heard to · utter the phrase "I'm bored." Indeed, the issue of "idleness," often associated with underemployment and typically identified as a source of youth dissatisfaction and crime in many slums and low income communities, was nonexistent for these young people.

The children of Sathyanagar had the advantage of being part of a generally cohesive culture steeped in tradition, myth and ritual that gave them a strong sense of identity. They knew who they were and had a strong sense of belonging due in part to their extended family networks, strong ties of kinship, and a vibrant social and cultural context in which

FIGURE 5. Children work individually or in pairs to take photographs of their area and their activities. They then work in small groups to share and discuss their photos as they begin to develop a common understanding of key issues and priorities for action. (Photo courtesy of S. R. Prakash)

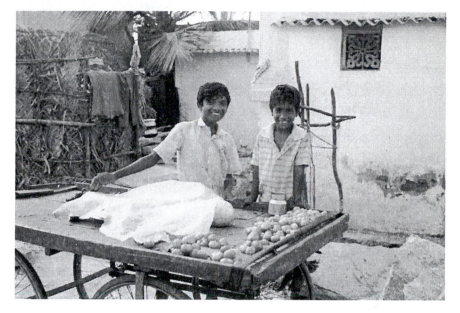

interaction with community members of all ages was an integral part of daily life. Religion and its symbols and rituals also played an important role in community life, as did diversity based upon language and place of origin.

Despite the environmental degradation caused by water pollution and inadequate sanitation and drainage, Sathyanagar contained a variety of spaces where the children could gather to play or to participate in community activities. There was a clear sense of community boundaries and a strong feeling of safety within the settlement itself (strengthened in no small measure by the lack of thru-traffic resulting from the community's location on a dead-end street). A glade of trees and small meadow in a ravine beside the railroad tracks, as well as the water and plants along the tank's edge, provided pockets of natural areas that were special places to many children, especially boys. Such a mosaic of accessible public and semi-public places has been identified to be critical for healthy child development (Bartlett et al., 1999; Cosco & Moore, 2002).

The children were keenly aware of the environmental problems and drawbacks of their local area, yet with few exceptions, their attitudes about the future were largely positive. Most children saw the community as having gotten better through their childhood years and on a path to further improvement. As one ten-year-old girl stated, "In the future, Sathyanagar will have a tap beside each house, and tarred roads. . . . It will be so good, they will write about us in the newspapers." When they were asked where they would like to live when they grew up, nearly all of the children who were interviewed did not hesitate in answering, "Sathyanagar."

## OBSTACLES TO YOUNG PEOPLE'S PARTICIPATION

While the stories shared by young people in Sathyanagar were infused with a grounded optimism about the future, their stories also told of first-hand experience with official neglect, broken promises, wasted resources and squandered opportunities, casting an unflattering light not only on inefficient, ineffective and sometimes inept or corrupt bureaucracies and politicians, but also on misguided development agencies and mismanaged nongovernmental groups (Driskell, Bannerjee & Chawla, 2001).

Although officially endorsed by the sponsoring agencies, and enshrined in the rhetoric of lead agency staff, the principles of 'community participation' in general, and young people's participation in particular, had little bearing on the way in which project proposals were developed or reviewed, the manner in which the lead organization was managed, or the way in which local decision makers understood and prioritized local issues.

As is too often the case in participation projects, the initial schedule of activities for the Bangalore Growing Up in Cities proposal–which had been purposely left open-ended to allow young people themselves to determine project outcomes–had to be rewritten to comply with the needs and priorities of potential funding agencies. This was an issue at several of the Growing Up in Cities sites–each of which had to raise its own funds to support local site activities. In Sathyanagar, the project's scope and budget had to be significantly expanded to be of interest to potential funders, incorporating a larger comprehensive planning effort and identifying specific project outcomes. Small projects with community-determined outcomes were seen as both risky and ineffective, requiring too much management effort by agency staff and too many challenges for ensuring accountability (accountability of the NGO to the funder, not to the community). Participatory research activities were also unsupportable, even if connected to subsequent (though as yet unspecified) implementation activities. Tangible, measurable outcomes (maps, plan documents, education materials, capital improvements) needed to be identified in the proposal. Community participation was of course paramount, but only as a vehicle for implementing pre-defined project outcomes.

Meaningful participation was further undermined by the dictatorial management of the lead program officer in the sponsoring NGO–who had voiced support for the principles of participation in community-based work, but found them irrelevant within the context of the organization. Local project staff members were regularly subjected to unilateral, unexplained decisions based on incomplete and often inaccurate information, as well as personal insults, degrading remarks about the quality of work being done, and regular threats of job termination. While local staff held up remarkably well under these circumstances, and retained their commitment to the project and the principles of participation, their efforts were ultimately cut short by the program manager's unilateral decision–motivated by a sense of being inadequately acknowledged and rewarded for her role in the project–to halt all work at the site, and end the NGO's involvement in the project. A significant amount of funding that had been raised on behalf of the community, and channeled through the NGO, was 'reassigned' to other, unspecified, uses. Project files, including data and maps that would be of significant value to the community, were locked in the NGO offices.

Although this decision was extremely upsetting, disruptive, and disrespectful to both the staff and the young participants, the responses from local staff members were indicative of the relationships they had developed in the community. Though several relied on their income from the NGO and did not want to jeopardize their employment, they had also developed a strong commitment to the project and to the young people in Sathyanagar. On their own initiative, they decided to continue the project work in their spare time. This made it possible to complete the remaining evaluation activities, and to identify and implement at least one of the priorities for improvement identified by young people in Sathyanagar: the need for a quiet place to study as well as a place for job training. In 1998, a Study Center was constructed by another NGO in the local area–one that had become increasingly involved in the project's work and demonstrated a commitment to child and youth participation. That NGO operated an informal school in the settlement, and was able to work with the project's core team to involve Sathyanagar's young people in the design and development process for the Study Center, which was constructed with funding provided by Norwegian children through the Norwegian Broadcasting Corporation's "Children's Hour" program.

Apart from these unanticipated internal obstacles to participation, the project also encountered the anticipated obstacles created by a system of political patronage, a fragmented bureaucracy, and corruption at nearly every level. The few politicians or bureaucrats who seemed to sincerely want to meet the needs of local young people were ill-equipped to do so in light of entrenched power relations and the complex bureaucracy. Perhaps most disheartening was the near complete lack of connection between what local officials viewed as the needs of local young people (more opportunities for sports and recreation) and what young people expressed as their needs (adequate clean water and sanitation). This inconsistency between official views of young people's needs, and young people's own perspectives on their needs, was a common characteristic among all the Growing Up in Cities sites. Also common was a general reluctance to engage young people in a participatory process of evaluation, planning and change, either because of the challenges that posed to current decision makers, or the belief that young people were not capable of understanding or contributing to the process of community development.

The experiences in Sathyanagar illustrate the obstacles faced by young people and disenfranchised communities when it comes to exercising their rights, including their right to define their own development priorities. They also raise fundamental issues about NGO ethics and accountability, and the all-too-common practice of the ends justifying the means. But it also achieved several important successes: the new Study Center was built; local staff developed an appreciation and skills for participatory methods; there was a noticeable shift in staff attitudes toward "slum" areas; and young people had a chance to think about the place where they lived and articulate their ideas about it (Figure 6). The research in Sathyanagar also gave insight into an area where much too little is known: the experience of poverty from children's perspectives. But the obstacles to young people's participation are significant, and very real.

FIGURE 6. Young people in Sathyanagar identified the need for a quiet place to study through the Growing Up in Cities project, and worked with a local NGO to develop this new study center in the settlement area. (Photo courtesy of David Driskell)

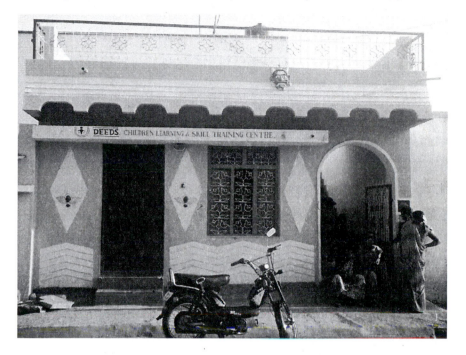

## COMPARING OUTCOMES

When Growing Up in Cities was introduced in Sathyanagar, its aim was not to demonstrate that top-down bureaucratic structures in aid agencies, nonprofit organizations and city planning offices thwart community participation. However, given a commitment to document both opportunities and obstacles to young people's inclusion in community planning, the project's outcomes included an analysis of these barriers, recommendations regarding ways that agencies can support genuine participation, and publications in media that would reach development planners (Driskell, Bannerjee & Chawla, 2001). One of the project's major operating principles is that people involved in initiatives of this kind need to learn from each other's successes and failures.

Nor did the project facilitators expect to find so many resources for children and youth in this marginal community. Sathyanagar, along with two communities in Argentina, came to be understood as examples of "paradoxical poverty"–places that were poor in material terms but rich in priceless social, cultural, and environmental advantages from young people's perspectives (see also Cosco & Moore, 2002; Lynch, 1977). To make this observation is not in any way to excuse all the people in positions of influence who could make conditions for families in these communities much better. Nevertheless, the story of Sathyanagar shows that one of the most important steps toward creating communities that serve young people's needs is to determine what is working well and to make it a priority to preserve and strengthen these assets. One of the reasons why young people's participation in community planning is vital is that nobody understands these assets better than young people themselves.

At the same time that research was underway in Sathyanagar, project sites were active in the United States, England and Australia (Malone & Hasluck, 2002; Percy-Smith, 2002; Salvadori, 2002). Despite much higher material standards of living, youth at these locations expressed acute levels of alienation. Another project outcome became a set of indicators of the characteristics that make a community a good place in which to grow up, or an alienating place, according to young people's own viewpoints. Although Growing Up in Cities has spanned a diverse range of cultures and urban conditions around the world, it has found remarkable consensus among young people with regard to these characteristics (Chawla, 2002). (See Figure 7.)

Fortunately, some of the project sites have been more successful than Sathyanagar at getting city officials' attention. This happened in a working-class suburb of Melbourne, Australia, where the project facilitators obtained the city council's commitment to engage young people as consultants in the redesign of a local park, and secured funding from Arts Victoria to bring a landscape designer into the local secondary school to help create a curriculum for community studies and to lead students through the collaborative creation of a new youth space for the park (Malone & Hasluck, 2002). Intrigued by a national radio story about the project, officials in neighboring Frankston invited the project facilitators to involve 8 through 18-year-olds in eight neighborhoods in assessing safety issues in their city. Participants' final recommendations were incorporated into the city's Safety Management Plan, and city councilors were so impressed by the usefulness of young people's ideas that they created a Youth Safety Management Team as an advisory body (Chawla & Malone, 2003). In Johannesburg, South Africa, initial project work with children in a squatter settlement attracted the

FIGURE 7. Indicators of Environmental Quality from Children's Perspectives. (Courtesy of UNESCO Publications and Louise Chawla)

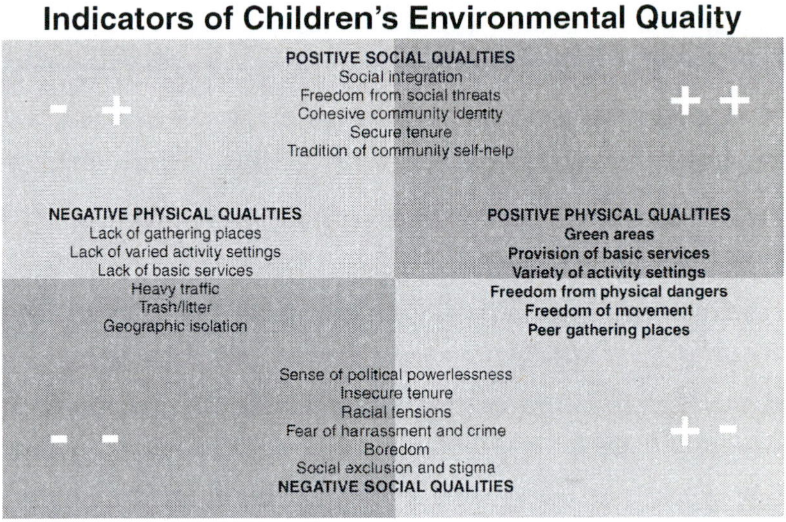

## Indicators of Children's Environmental Quality

**POSITIVE SOCIAL QUALITIES**
Social integration
Freedom from social threats
Cohesive community identity
Secure tenure
Tradition of community self-help

**NEGATIVE PHYSICAL QUALITIES**
Lack of gathering places
Lack of varied activity settings
Lack of basic services
Heavy traffic
Trash/litter
Geographic isolation

**POSITIVE PHYSICAL QUALITIES**
Green areas
Provision of basic services
Variety of activity settings
Freedom from physical dangers
Freedom of movement
Peer gathering places

Sense of political powerlessness
Insecure tenure
Racial tensions
Fear of harrassment and crime
Boredom
Social exclusion and stigma
**NEGATIVE SOCIAL QUALITIES**

attention of the Mayor, Isaac Mogase, who invited the children to present their evaluation of their settlement and their visions for a better life to high-ranking city officials (Kruger & Chawla, 2002). Subsequently, the Greater Johannesburg Metropolitan Council commissioned the project director in South Africa to organize a series of workshops with children in four city districts, and these, in turn, became the model for a series of workshops to enable young people to express their views on the issues that they face in the surrounding Gauteng Province (Kruger & Chawla, 2002). Official action in response to the four-site report was derailed by a change in administration, but a follow-up study commissioned by Save the Children Sweden to investigate the lack of action has prompted a renewed commitment to put the young people's ideas to use (Clements, 2003).

## *PARTNERSHIPS FOR COMMUNITY CHANGE*

A survey of all the reports that have been sent to UNESCO from Growing Up in Cities sites around the world point to the following general conclusions:

1. Adult decision makers usually do not have an accurate understanding of young people's issues and priorities.
2. Even young children can engage in a meaningful evaluation of their community and offer realistic recommendations for community change. (The youngest Growing Up in Cities participants have been eight years old, but when projects focus on nearby environments, even younger children can contribute in significant ways.)
3. The most effective model for achieving change involves children, youth and adults *working together* to ensure that young people's voices are heard and that they have a role in influencing the decisions that affect their lives.

Achieving meaningful change requires that adults not only reach out to young people and treat them as partners in the community development process, but also that they work together to develop a network of adult allies who have the necessary resources, political clout, and commitment to help young people turn their ideas into reality. One paramount rule, all project facilitators agree, is, "Network, network, network."

Another important lesson that has stood out is that putting young people at the center of community development has been an effective approach for promoting human-centered development in general. Community leaders, government officials, and others in position of power (including parents) are more willing to work together to make change happen if they see evidence that it will improve young people's lives.

Although small in scale, Growing Up in Cities has been an effective global demonstration of the active role that young people can play in community change processes–not just in the resource-rich countries of the global North, or in communities of privilege, but also in the developing countries of the global South and in communities that have been traditionally marginalized and lacking in financial resources. It shows that when adults in influence are prepared to not just listen to young people but *hear* them and take their ideas seriously, the bold principles set forth in the Convention on the Rights of the Child can be implemented in practice.

## NOTES

1. Ironically, the United States brought the civil rights clauses to the table when the Convention on the Rights of the Child was being drafted, but now the United States and Somalia stand alone as the only member states of the United Nations which have not yet ratified the Convention. Nevertheless, as the most widely ratified human rights

treaty in history, the Convention is considered to have assumed the universal status of customary law.

2. As a signatory to the Habitat Agenda, the United States has committed itself to this goal of including children and youth in community planning.

3. For more information about the project, see www.unesco.org/most/growing.htm.

4. For a more extensive description of the project's methods and findings, see Driskell and Bannerjee (2002).

# REFERENCES

Bannerjee, K., & Driskell, D. (2002). Tales from Truth Town. In L. Chawla (Ed.), *Growing up in an urbanising world* (pp. 135-160). London/Paris: Earthscan Publications/UNESCO.

Bartlett, S., Hart, R., Satterthwaite, D., De la Barra, X., & Missair, A. (1999). *Cities for children*. London/New York: Earthscan Publications/UNICEF.

Chawla, L. (Ed.). (2002). *Growing up in an urbanising world*. London/Paris: Earthscan Publications/UNESCO.

Chawla, L., & Malone, K. (2003). Neighborhood quality in children's eyes. In P. Christensen & M. O'Brien (Eds.), *Children in the city* (pp. 118-141). London: Routledge-Falmer.

Clements, J. (2003). How crazy can it be? An assessment, three years later, of outcomes from a participatory project with children in Johannesburg. Oslo: Save the Children Sweden. Retrieved March 2, 2005 from http://www.colorado.edu/journals/cye/14_1/workinprogress/

Cosco, N., & Moore, R. (2002). "Our neighborhood is like that!" Cultural richness and childhood identity in Boca-Barracas, Buenos Aires. In L. Chawla (Ed.), *Growing up in an urbanising world* (pp. 35-56). London/Paris: Earthscan Publications/UNESCO.

Driskell, D. (2002). *Creating better cities with children and youth*. London/Paris: Earthscan Publications/UNESCO.

Driskell, D., Bannerjee, K., & Chawla, L. (2001). Rhetoric, reality and resilience: Overcoming obstacles to young people's participation in development. *Environment and Urbanization, 13* (1), 77-89.

Hart, R. (1997). *Children's participation: The theory and practice of involving young citizens in community development and environmental care*. London/New York: Earthscan Publications/UNICEF.

Kruger, J., & Chawla, L. (2002). "We know something someone doesn't know . . . " Children speak out on local conditions in Johannesburg. *Environment and Urbanization, 14*(2): 85-96.

Lynch, K. (Ed.) (1977). *Growing up in cities*. Cambridge, MA: MIT Press.

Malone, K., & Hasluck, L. (2002). Australian youth. In L. Chawla (Ed.), *Growing up in an urbanizing world* (pp. 81-109). London/Paris: Earthscan Publications/UNESCO.

Percy-Smith, B. (2002). Contested worlds. In L. Chawla (Ed.), *Growing up in an urbanising world* (pp. 57-80). London/Paris: Earthscan Publications/UNESCO.

Salvadori, I. (2002). Between fences. In L. Chawla (Ed.), *Growing up in an urbanizing world* (pp. 183-200). London/Paris: Earthscan Publications/Paris.

Swart-Kruger, J. (2002). Children in a South African squatter camp gain and lose a voice. In L. Chawla (Ed.), *Growing up in an urbanising world* (pp. 111-133).

United Nations. (1989). *Convention on the Rights of the Child.* Retrieved April 2, 2005 from www.unicef.org/crc/crc.htm

United Nations Centre for Human Settlements. (1996). *The Habitat Agenda.* Nairobi: UNCHS. Retrieved April 2, 2005 from www.unchs.org/unchs/english/hagenda/index.htm

# STUDENT FACILITATORS
# AND COLLABORATIVE TEAMS
# FOR PARTICIPATION

## Training Students as Facilitators in the Youth Empowerment Strategies (YES!) Project

Nance Wilson, PhD
Meredith Minkler, DrPH
Stefan Dasho, MA
Roxanne Carrillo, MSW
Nina Wallerstein, DrPH
Diego Garcia, AA

Nance Wilson is Co-Investigator and Program Director, Youth Empowerment Strategies (*YES!*), Public Health Institute, Berkeley, CA. Meredith Minkler is *YES!* Project Collaborator/Consultant; Professor, University of California, School of Public Health, Division of Community Health and Human Development, Berkeley, CA. Stefan Dasho is *YES!* Program Evaluator, Public Health Institute, Berkeley, CA. Roxanne Carrillo is *YES!* Project Collaborator; Manager, Healthy Neighborhoods Project, Public Health Collaborations Unit, Public Health Division, Contra Costa Health Services, CA. Nina Wallerstein is *YES!* Project Co-investigator; Professor, Masters in Public Health Program, University of New Mexico, Albuquerque, NM. Diego Garcia is affiliated with Art Instruction and *YES!* Project Collaborator; Afterschool Program Coordinator, Grant Elementary School, Richmond, CA.

Address correspondence to: Nance Wilson, Youth Empowerment Strategies, Public Health Institute, 2140 Shattuck Avenue, Suite #401, Berkeley, CA 94704 (E-mail: nwilson@phi.org).

This research was supported by Grant No. R06/CCR921439-01 from the Centers for Disease Control and Prevention. The opinions expressed in this paper do not necessarily reflect the views of the funding agency.

[Haworth co-indexing entry note]: "Training Students as Facilitators in the Youth Empowerment Strategies (YES!) Project." Wilson, Nance et al. Co-published simultaneously in *Journal of Community Practice* (The Haworth Press, Inc.) Vol. 14, No. 1/2, 2006, pp. 201-217; and: *Youth Participation and Community Change* (ed: Barry N. Checkoway, and Lorraine M. Gutiérrez) The Haworth Press, Inc., 2006, pp. 201-217. Single or multiple copies of this article are available for a fee from The Haworth Document Delivery Service [1-800-HAWORTH, 9:00 a.m. - 5:00 p.m. (EST). E-mail address: docdelivery@haworthpress.com].

**SUMMARY.** This article describes the training of students as facilitators for the Youth Empowerment Strategies (YES!) project designed to promote problem-solving, social action and civic participation among underserved elementary school youth in West Contra Costa County, California. This project involved 160 fifth grade students in after-school activities which identified their capacities and strengths in ways which aimed to decrease rates of alcohol, tobacco and other drug use and other risky behaviors. The article describes the recruitment and training of high school students and their graduate student counterparts as facilitators in this university-community partnership, and discusses the implications for other youth-focused community-based projects. *[Article copies available for a fee from The Haworth Document Delivery Service: 1-800-HAWORTH. E-mail address: <docdelivery@haworthpress.com> Website: <http://www.HaworthPress.com> © 2006 by The Haworth Press, Inc. All rights reserved.]*

**KEYWORDS.** University-community partnership, community-based participatory research, adolescent health, prevention, after school programs, Photovoice

## INTRODUCTION

Continued high rates of alcohol, tobacco and other drug use (ATOD) in youth, coupled with risky behaviors that can lead to HIV/AIDS, teen pregnancy and other problematic outcomes (Futterman, Chabon, & Hoffman, 2000; Resnick et al., 1997; Sanders-Phillips, 1996; Whaley, 1999; Wilson, Battistich, Syme, & Boyce, 2002), have led practitioners and researchers to look for new and innovative ways of studying and addressing these complex problems (Kirby, 2001; Sanders-Phillips, 1996; Wallerstein, Sanchez-Merki, & Dow, 2005; Whaley, 1999). Increasingly, these new approaches have involved academic-community partnerships in which local youth become an integral part of the research and intervention team (Blaine et al., 1997; Cheatham & Shen, 2003; Tencati, Kole, Feigher, Winkleby, & Altman, 2002). Although most often in such partnerships, the academic or professional partners determine the issues to be investigated and addressed (Reason, 1994; Stoecker, 1999), a promising new approach is gaining increasing popularity, and involves creating the conditions in which youth become empowered to study and act on issues that they themselves identify (Cheatham & Shen, 2003; Wallerstein, 2002; Wallerstein, Larson-Bright,

Adams, & Rael, 2000). An example of such an approach is Youth Empowerment Strategies (*YES!*), a CDC-funded Community Based Participatory Prevention Research (CBPR) project designed to promote problem-solving skills, social action and civic participation among underserved elementary school youth in West Contra Costa County (WCCC), California (Grant No. R06/CCR921439-01). Although the outcome goals of this three year project include decreasing rates of alcohol, tobacco and other drug (ATOD) use and other risky behaviors, the program does not focus directly on such problems, but rather involves a strengths-based approach (Saleeby, 1997). *YES!* builds on the existing capacities of youth in these low income neighborhoods, and helps them develop the tools needed to identify, study and address issues of shared concern on the school, neighborhood and larger community levels. This paper will describe and critically analyze the recruitment and training of local high school students and their graduate student counterparts for their roles as the facilitators in a unique after school program. Implications and recommendations for other academic-community partnerships involving youth-focused CBPR projects will be discussed.

## WEST CONTRA COSTA COUNTY

The urban neighborhoods of WCCC confront a plethora of problems including high rates of substance abuse, crime, unemployment, toxic waste, and HIV/AIDS, and large pockets of poverty (American FactFinder, 2000; Walker, Brunner, Wise, & Leivermann, 2003). Youth in this geographic area are similarly challenged, having both high rates of teen births (State of California Master Birth File 1991-1999) and the highest drop out rates in Contra Costa County. West County's homicide rate is one of the highest in the United States; from 1991 through 2001, homicide was the leading cause of death for youth aged of 15 and 19. They attend schools which score at the bottom of the state Academic Placement Index and the California Fitness Test (School Accountability Report Card School Year 2000-2001). Despite these troubling realities, however, an asset-based approach to this locality reveals multi-ethnic neighborhoods rich in both cultural and civic organizations, and with a tradition of organizing and community building around toxic chemical spills and other problems (Community Health Assessment Planning and Evaluation Unit, 2003; El-Askari et al., 1998; Minkler, 2000). These assets and strengths were drawn upon in the mid 1990s when the local health department catalyzed the "Healthy Neighborhoods Project"

(HNP). Using a community organizing and community building approach, the HNP forged a strong partnership between local residents, community based organizations, and the local health department. Ten resident community organizers and 120 Neighborhood Health Advocates were trained in neighborhood asset and risk mapping, basic survey research and other methods which they then used with youth and other residents in helping them to identify shared concerns and mobilize to help address them. Working in several neighborhoods, the HNP counted among its victories getting evening bus service restored; increasing activities for youth; forming a local "bucket brigade" to monitor air pollution; and convening youth, adults, police and city officials to reduce tensions and plan long term violence prevention strategies (Community Health Assessment Planning and Evaluation Unit, 2003; El-Askari et al., 1998; Minkler, 2000). The HNP and Contra Costa Health Services are a *YES!* program ally, contributing to current and future plans for the program and to the training of the co-facilitators.

The conceptual risk model (Figure 1) upon which *YES!* is based states that individuals living in distressed neighborhoods have higher levels of exposure to physical and environmental disorder (e.g., brown fields, abandoned buildings and vacant lots), and to social disorder (ranging from harassment to violence). According to the model, this increased exposure leads to negative changes in beliefs and attitudes, which in turn result in decreased health-promoting behaviors. In adults, outcome measures would include chronic diseases (e.g., cardiovascular disease, diabetes, etc.). In young adolescents, the outcomes are markers for later health outcomes, and include violence, ATOD use, early school leaving, anti-social behaviors, unwanted pregnancy, exposure to HIV/AIDS, depression, and other such health and social outcomes.

The *YES!* intervention model (Figure 2) posits that participation in *YES!* groups influences positively behaviors and beliefs (e.g., future orientation, individual and group efficacy, perceived influence) which, in turn, positively influences proximal outcomes, as evidenced by changes in conflict resolution skills, group collaborative decision-making, and agentic behavior, ultimately resulting in increased health and wellness outcomes. Although these models are presented as linear, they are interactive.

*YES!* has adapted many elements of the earlier Adolescent Social Action Program (ASAP) in Albuquerque, New Mexico. Operating from the early 1980s through the late 1990s, ASAP was a youth-centered empowerment model prevention program that was implemented in over 30 middle and high schools in vulnerable neighborhoods. The goals of ASAP

## FIGURE 1. The *YES!* Conceptual Risk Model

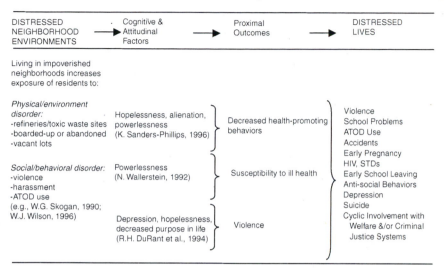

centered on reducing morbidity and mortality, encouraging youth to make healthier choices, and using empowerment education to actively engage youth in social and political action in their schools and neighborhoods (Dow-Velarde, Starling, & Wallerstein, 2002; Wallerstein et al., 2005). ASAP, in short, modeled the strengths-based empowerment approach that is central to the *YES!* program. ASAP's intergenerational approach, in which graduate and undergraduate college students were trained as facilitators for an empowerment model after school program for early adolescents, forms a central core of the *YES!* approach. Although evaluation of the ASAP program proved challenging, in part because tools and measures for gauging change through empowerment programs are still in their infancy, program intervention youth were shown to have a number of statistically significant increases in areas such as self-efficacy around protecting family and friends, empathy, and social influence or perceived control. Broader level changes also were observed, with ASAP youth linking with other efforts (e.g., a gang prevention project and a statewide youth policy development project) to address shared concerns (Wallerstein et al., 2005).

As noted above, the *YES!* project builds in part on ASAP but incorporates the *Photovoice* method developed by Caroline Wang (Wang, 2003; Wang & Burris, 1994). The *Photovoice* approach provides community members with cameras and training in how to use them in order to take pic-

FIGURE 2. The *YES!* Intervention Model

| EMPOWERMENT PROCESS $\rightarrow$ | Cognitive & Attitudinal $\rightarrow$ Factors | Proximal Empowerment $\rightarrow$ Outcomes | HEALTH & WELLNESS OUTCOMES |
|---|---|---|---|

| *Participation in YES! Groups:* | | -Use of collaborative decision-making* | *Increased:* |
| *Photovoice*, dialogue-reflection-action and other PAR approaches | Future Orientation˙ | -Use of conflict resolution skills* | -Awareness of risky behaviors+ -Health-promoting behaviors+ |
| | Social Cohesion˙ | | |
| School Social Action Project | Measures of Personal and Group Efficacy˙ | -Increased involvement in designing and implementing positive project efforts* | *Reduced:* |
| Neighborhood Social Action Project | Perceived Influence˙ | | ATOD use+ Accidents+ |
| Community Social Action Project | | -Increased efficacy and political participation* | Anti-social behaviors+ Decreased violence+ Depression+ |

˙Quantitative measures; *Qualitative observation

tures that convey their "images of the world," including both the strengths and the problems experienced in their local communities. Under the leadership of a trained facilitator, the pictures are used to generate group dialogue during which participants discuss their pictures often using the mnemonic SHOWeD (Shaffer, 1983). What do you *S*ee here? What's really *H*appening here? How does this relate to *O*ur lives? What can we *D*o about it? Formation and implementation of an action plan is a central part of the *Photovoice* method, which has been used effectively with diverse groups, such as inner-city youth (Strack & Magill, 2004), homeless people (Wang, 2003), and rural women in China (Wang, Yi, Tao, & Carovano, 1998). Previous successful use of *Photovoice* by the Contra Costa Health Services, Division of Maternal Child Health (Spears, 1999) underscored its local relevance and utility. There are several other significant differences between ASAP and *YES!*, including program duration (six weeks compared to three years), age group (middle and high school compared to elementary school), and importantly, thanks to the nature of the CDC/CBPR funding, *YES!* was able to design an intervention that was not targeted specifically to ATOD-related topics. As suggested later, this funding flexibility enabled *YES!* participants to develop potential social action projects in a wide range of areas of concern to youth, and reflected the CBPR principle of community-driven issue selection. In sum, the *YES!* project model was well-grounded in earlier empowerment intervention efforts and has partnered with key individuals from these programs to help in the design, training and implementation of the new model. It also uniquely tailored the intervention model to the strengths and needs of children in WCCC.

## THE YES! PROGRAM

The *YES!* intervention is a three-year after school program based on the principles of individual and community empowerment and capacity building (Wallerstein, 1992; Zimmerman, 2000), and community based participatory research (Castelloe, Watson, & White, 2002; Israel, Schulz, Parker, & Becker, 1998; Yosihama & Carr, 2002). *YES!* program staff, who conceptualized and direct the project, operate out of a bridging organization, the Oakland-based Public Health Institute (PHI), which is known for its history of innovative work linking academia with health departments and local community partners. Through sub-contracts with PHI, *YES!* creates an academic partnership involving faculty and graduate students at the University of California, Berkeley, the University of New Mexico, Albuquerque, and the local health department (HNP) with a community partnership including high school students and local public schools. The goal of the *YES!* program is to help vulnerable children have healthy, fulfilling lives and a sense of hope for the future. We hypothesize that children's active involvement in participatory approaches to social action will help them develop a stronger future orientation, while helping to create a sense of cohesion, efficacy, and perceived influence over their world. We further believe that having a sense of future will promote healthy behaviors, as well as increase children's awareness of some behaviors as healthy or as risky. As noted above, the program's focus is not directly on changing risk behaviors, but rather on enhancing the strengths and capacities of the children as they transition into adolescence and into middle school (Wilson et al., 2003).

Funded in the fall of 2002, the *YES!* program provided intensive initial training to high school and college graduate student pairs. By winter, 2003, the co-facilitator pairs were working in the *YES!* after school program at four elementary schools. Ten groups of 5th graders each used *Photovoice*, community asset and risk mapping (Brown, 2003; McKnight & Kretzmann, 1990), and other techniques to design a social action project in their "school community." In year two (6th grade) the focus will continue to be the school community and may expand to the students' local neighborhoods, then in year three (7th grade), each student group will identify a local community leader or elder with whom it would like to undertake a social action project.

## Facilitator Recruitment

Given the above goals, careful attention was paid to the recruitment and training of the facilitators, since their role is critical for building group cohesion, prompting critical dialogue and shepherding the social action. Unlike ASAP, the *YES!* project paired high school students (community partners) as co-facilitators with graduate students (academic partners). The purpose of including high school students in *YES!* was to be able to draw on their knowledge of the community and of local youth culture and thus better tailor the program contextually. In year one of this project, seven high school students from the WCCC Unified School District and six graduate students from the University of California, Berkeley were recruited and trained to work as paid co-facilitators in the *YES!* project. Community partners associated with several elementary and high schools, including after school program coordinators, academic advisors and other school personnel helped the project staff to locate these high school students. A similarly wide net was cast to recruit the graduate students through professors, fellow students and postings.

Recruitment considerations included experience working with children in a community organizing, mentoring or teaching capacity, as well as having a future orientation (e.g., goals and future plans after high school), critical thinking skills (e.g., ability to imagine multiple causality for student motivation), and a non-punitive orientation to behavior management (reflected, for example, in their response to the question "What would you do if a group participant appeared to be taking the group intentionally off-task by acting out?"). These characteristics (sense of future, critical thinking and positive orientation to behavior management/conflict resolution) were considered important to model for the *YES!* group participants. An emphasis also was placed on finding students of diverse racial/ethnic backgrounds, reflecting the diversity of the elementary school-aged populations being served. In addition to learning about candidates' past experiences and future goals, potential co-facilitators were asked questions that would help reveal their leadership skills and cultural and other sensitivities. For example, they were asked how they might respond to specific situations in a group session, e.g., "what would you do if someone made a racist remark or put down?" The recruited group of co-facilitators was highly diverse along multiple dimensions and several were bicultural and bilingual, with five languages spoken in all.

## Facilitator Training: Goals and Approach

The majority of the 60-hour facilitator training took place over a period of five weeks, mostly in full-day weekend sessions, with additional "practice" and discussion sessions. The goals of the training for the participants included: (1) understanding the rationale and goals of the project, (2) experiencing program processes first hand (e.g., dialogue and *Photovoice*), (3) learning facilitation and group management skills, (4) understanding expectations for the content of the first weeks of sessions and (5) developing a comfort level and skill in working collaboratively with a co-facilitator. A variety of academic and community partners from diverse racial/ethnic backgrounds and areas of expertise were involved as trainers over the course of the training program. The *YES!* training emphasized four major tools: empowerment education, *Photovoice*, community action and participatory research, and cooperative learning. In Table 1, the actual topics presented are grouped according to their purpose.

Most of the training sessions combined several elements: experience with group development tools, the rationale and conceptual underpinnings for the use of tools, both in terms of project goals and child development, presenters' practical advice about implementation and opportunities to reflect on and debrief the session. (The training manual is available upon request, Dasho & Wilson, 2002.) The iterative nature of the training deserves some comment, since this term is used frequently to suggest that adjustments and refinements of staff development content and processes have been made along the way, based on need or feedback. As in other participatory action research (Alvarez & Gutiérrez, 2001), the particular mix of strategies and components that comprised the *YES!* training truly evolved as an outgrowth of collaboration and experimentation. As will be discussed later, this resulted in ongoing staff development and curriculum creation on a scale equivalent to the initial training sessions.

## Self-Assessments of Preparedness

Following the final training session, all facilitators rated themselves "well prepared" overall to lead their groups; however, several of the graduate students reported that they wouldn't feel they knew the community until they began to work there. Similarly, some of the high school students indicated a lack of confidence in leading some of the facilitation strategies, such as SHOWeD discussion and forum building. In short, and despite an overall sense of readiness and preparedness for their roles as facilitators, there was considerable intra-group variation in preparedness regarding diversity issues, photography and group management. When interviewed after groups had met for two months, facilitators noted that the biggest discrepancies with their initial expectations were difficulties engaging students in discussion and determining whether students understood concepts the facilitators had presented. As one graduate student reported: "It's challenging to rethink things for the 5th grade level. I need to focus on what is really important for students to learn in each session so that we have a sense of the priority for using the time and to develop relationships that will help them be productive." Another high school student commented: "Because we were well prepared I thought we would be able to just walk in and do it but it is messier dealing with real situations and it is harder to recover when things go wrong. You think it is going to go smoothly but it doesn't."

As the groups entered their third month working together, each had its own unique character. While the facilitators in some groups grappled with highly distractible students, other facilitators were trying to find ways to get extremely quiet students to participate in discussions. Despite these group-specific challenges, facilitators appeared to have a common need for much more explicit direction in creating the agenda for each session, resulting in the development of the detailed weekly curriculum guides discussed below.

### Curriculum Development and Initial Outcomes

Project staff initially assumed that the groups would proceed at their own pace. It soon became clear, however, that all groups would benefit from detailed, week by week curriculum guides designed to get the groups to the point where they would design their social action project. Some facilitators were uncomfortable selecting activities themselves, while others had difficulty allocating time to address the most important priorities for a session. Despite the desire to be sensitive to the unique strengths and needs of each group, some curriculum standardization was desirable in order to: (1) further information exchange between and among project staff and facilitators, (2) pilot and refine activities for the development of a training manual, and (3) enable subsequent replication of the intervention. As facilitators noted: "I appreciate the lesson plans; even though I was used to doing my own as a teacher, a lot has to go into creating these activities." "I'm happy with *YES!*'s responsiveness when [a facilitator] put[s] out need for more direction. I feel I am

## TABLE 1. Training Topics and Approaches

| Purpose | Specific Training Topics | Session Presenters and Resources |
|---|---|---|
| Working with children in West Contra Costa County | Community challenges & health issues | Chuck McKetney, Ph.D., Community Health Assessment & Evaluation, Contra Costa Health Services |
| | Multicultural awareness | Afriye Quamina, Ed.D.: Experiential exercises on interpersonal communication & authority |
| Working with children | Child development & protection issues | Carrie Frazier, M.S.W.: Stages of development (Erikson, 1963); legal and counseling implications of abuse |
| Community action and participatory research | Neighborhood issues & community forum building; asset & risk mapping | Roxanne Carrillo, M.S.W., and Mr. Sari Tatpaporn, HNP, Contra Costa Health Services (McKnight, 1990) |
| | Community organizing | Meredith Minkler, Dr.PH, UC Berkeley (Minkler, 2004) |
| Group facilitation | Intrinsic motivation, group management, teambuilding, group decision-making | Stefan Dasho, M.A., *YES!* project: Expanding the Developmental Discipline approach (Watson, 2003) |
| Empowerment education | Freirian dialogue | Nina Wallerstein, Dr.PH, UNM, Albuquerque: Modeling critical dialogue (Wallerstein et al., in press) |
| | *Photovoice* | Lisa S. Powers: *Photovoice* experience (Wang, 1998) |
| | Choosing themes | Eveline Shen & Ann Cheatham (APIRH): Modeling theme selection |
| | Writing and empowerment | Alma Flor Ada, Ph.D., & F. Isabel Campoy: Writing for empowerment (Ada & Campoy, 2004) |
| Project specific information | Confidentiality & project goals | Nance Wilson, Ph.D., & Stefan Dasho, M.A., *YES!* project |

self-critical and when we recognize a problem we have tried to figure out solutions." "I didn't expect curriculum, which is both good and bad. The lessons don't address the differences in the groups but make the sessions easier to do."

To create the curriculum the program evaluator and the program director visited all groups to assess both group needs and progress. Facilitators needed more than monthly staff meetings to understand the purpose of the activities, so individual weekly conference times were set up to discuss the upcoming lesson plans with each graduate student. This arrangement reflected the easy access of the graduate students to the project office, and the difficulty of arranging time, other than during the group sessions, to meet with the high school students. It also acknowledged the reality that the graduate students clearly took the lead in each of the groups, despite both the "egalitarian" model of "co-facilitation" presented in the training, and the graduate students' efforts to share responsibility. In the second year, to assist in status equalization between the academic and community co-facilitation partners, the project initiated group meetings with high school students provide them with a forum for expressing their experience and facilitation needs as well as to have advance preparation for the curriculum.

The curriculum was designed to cover four domains: teambuilding, photography, activities using empowerment education processes, and developing a social action project. Given the mid-year start of the program, the curriculum was designed to introduce all four domains in 13 sessions. At that point, the groups would determine their social action projects and carry them out over the remaining weeks of school. Teambuilding and photography were emphasized during the first half of the 13 weeks while the second half focused on photography as a trigger for critical dialogue and identification of the assets and issues that would be the subject of the social action project. (The curriculum is available upon request, Dasho & Wilson, 2003.) When the groups in the first two schools were in their seventh week of sessions, groups at the two other schools began. It was possible to revise the curriculum based on a review of student evaluations, co-facilitator session logs, observation of 90% of the sessions by the project staff, and meetings with the co-facilitators to provide feedback on the curriculum. This is in keeping with the principles of participatory research and of academic-community partnerships, demonstrating the bi-directionality of the learning that took place (Anderson, 2002; Castelloe et al., 2002; Israel et al., 1998; Yosihama & Carr, 2002).

By the end of the school year, all ten groups had consensually agreed upon a social action project and had completed some aspect of that project. Predictably the groups which started late were able to do less in the realm of community action than the groups which had more time, and instead developed photobooks or posters or made presentations to their schools. In contrast, the groups which got an earlier start developed projects which included designing, administering and tabulating surveys on graffiti and mural replacement, organizing cleanups, getting first aid instruction and doing petition drives to get sports back into physical education and pledges to participate in school beautification. Ongoing group observation and student interviews at the end of the school year revealed that a genuine bonding between members occurred in six of the ten groups. Three of the four groups that did not exhibit or report cohesiveness were late starting groups. All students reported feeling pride and excitement about using cameras. Interviews conducted by project staff at the end of the school year revealed this aspect of the project to be the most rewarding from the students' perspective. The hiatus imposed by the long summer break, which occurred for several groups soon after topic selection, resulted in some loss of momentum and changes in interest areas. However, many of the initial social action processes demonstrated group creativity and planning skills, and laid important ground work for the second year.

## IMPLICATIONS FOR PRACTICE

Although the *YES!* project is in its first year of operation, the experiences to date in training a core group of college and high school student facilitators suggest a number of implications for others interested in training youth empowerment workers through an academic-community partnership model. First, "cookbook recipes" for activities are neither adequate nor desirable. As the *YES!* project team learned, facilitators need to understand each session's intended purpose, what the participants should be able to walk away with from each activity, and what the relative priorities should be among the various objectives of the session. The lesson plans highlighted session objectives and desired outcomes so that facilitators could modify lessons to maximize the impact of each activity. Facilitators did not appear to feel confident with this, however, and tended to try to "get through" a lesson. Second, while it is helpful to discuss a generic "toolkit" of facilitation strategies during the training, facilitators may prefer to have specific tools attached to each activity. For example, we revised the lesson plans to designate a participation strategy such as "have partners brainstorm ideas" or "go around the circle having each student offer one idea at a time" rather than expect facilitators to think of one on their own.

Another implication for practice is that children at this age require physical movement and play. A balance must be struck between work and play in order to ensure motivation and attention, and accomplishing needed tasks. Facilitator training needs to include ways of helping to strike this balance. Moreover, in today's school cultures, students frequently become accustomed to receiving rewards for doing their work. Youth empowerment projects face the difficulty of balancing (or tipping the balance of) extrinsic and intrinsic motivation (Deci & Ryan, 1991). Facilitator training should include ample time for dialogue about the difference between using snacks, pizza parties and playtime as celebrations of accomplishments vs. using these treats as behavior-contingent rewards which can undermine the goal of self motivation.

Whether they are academic or community partners, it is a challenge for facilitators in an after school program to establish authority in a way that both maintains control and encourages participants' empowerment, which often lead to group management issues. Specifically, the majority of the facilitators seemed conflicted with the role of being "an authority" and instead tried to be "pals" with the student participants. Several expressed concern that they didn't know how to keep students in line without using the threat of a consequence for misbehavior. This tension would appear to be not so much a lack of experience as it is a concern about violating "empowerment" approaches. A significant amount of ongoing discussion focused on task engagement and techniques for intervening when students were disruptive. The most common strategies used were to remind them of the rules and to have one co-facilitator take them aside to problem-solve what was occurring. Over time these strategies proved somewhat effective with most students. However, leaders of empowerment groups must continually grapple with the decision to continue to work with or "dis-invite" disruptive students. Finally, preparing high school and graduate students as co-facilitators underscored the importance of responding flexibly to unique dynamics of each group. Once again the importance of balance is emphasized, with attention both to slowing down to achieve a depth in understanding session objectives and moving on if the participants have clearly indicated that they need a break or a fresh approach.

## CONCLUSION

The YES! project offers a theory-driven intervention, grounded in principles of empowerment and participatory research, and based on an academic-community partnership approach. Critical to the notion of praxis is the fact that the learning comes about through the undertaking of action. Our understanding of what it takes to prepare facilitators to implement empowerment education strategies at the elementary school level was shaped in the spirit of co-learning that characterizes both CBPR efforts and academic community partnerships (Anderson, 2002; Green et al., 1995; Israel et al., 1998; Yosihama & Carr, 2002). This organizational learning centered upon meeting the needs of facilitators for clarity of purpose, structure and freedom and support in group management. The lessons learned suggest that other academic partners in health education, social work and related fields who are interested in the design and implementation of empowerment projects with youth need to proactively enable this type of co-learning.

# REFERENCES

Ada, A.F., & Campoy, F.I. (2003). *Authors in the classroom: A transformative education process.* Boston: Pearson.

Alvarez, A.R., & Gutiérrez, L.M. (2001). Choosing to do participatory research: An example and issues of fit to consider. *Journal of Community Practice, 9*(1). 1-21.

American FactFinder. (2000). *Profile of selected economic characteristics, Richmond City, California.* Retrieved June 30, 2003, from http://www.factfinder.census.gov

Anderson, S. (2002). Engaging students in community-based research: A model for teaching social work research. *Journal of Community Practice, 10*(2), 71-87.

Blaine, T.M., Forster, J.L., Hennrikus, D., O'Neil, S., Wolfson, M., & Pham, H. (1997). Creating tobacco control policy at the local level: Implementation of a direct action approach. *Health Education and Behavior, 24*(5), 640-651.

Brown, M.P. (2003). Risk mapping as a tool for community based participatory research and organizing (pp. 446-450). In M. Minkler & N. Wallerstein (Eds.), *Community based participatory research for health.* San Francisco: Jossey-Bass.

Castelloe, P., Watson, W., & White, C. (2002). Participatory change: An integrative approach to community practice. *Journal of Community Practice, 10*(4), 7-31.

Cheatham, A., & Shen, E. (2003). Community based participatory research with Cambodian girls in Long Beach, California (pp. 316-331). In M. Minkler & N. Wallerstein (Eds.), *Community based participatory research for health.* San Francisco: Jossey-Bass.

Community Health Assessment Planning and Evaluation Unit, Health Services Department. (2003). Analysis of state of California death statistical master file. Martinez: Contra Costa County, Health Services Department.

Dasho, S., & Wilson, N. (2002). *Empowering youth: Facilitator manual.* Youth Empowerment Strategies Project. (Unpublished manuscript)

Dasho, S., & Wilson, N. (2003). *Youth Empowerment Strategies curriculum guide.* Youth Empowerment Strategies Project. (Unpublished manuscript)

Deci, E., & Ryan, R.M. (1991). A motivational approach to self: Integration in personality. In R. Dienstbier (Ed.), *Nebraska symposium on motivation, Volume 38: Perspectives on Motivation.* University of Nebraska Press.

Dow-Velarde, L., Starling, R., & Wallerstein, N. (2002). Social action for adolescent prevention. In T.M. Brinthaupt & R.P. Lipka (Eds.), *Understanding the self in the early adolescent* (pp. 267-291). NY: University of New York State Press.

DuRant, R.H., Cadenhead, C., Pendergast, R.A., Slaven, G., & Linder, C.W. (1994). Factors associated with the use of violence among urban Black adolescents. *American Journal of Public Health, 84,* 612-617.

El-Askari, G., Freestone, J., Irizarry, C., Kraut, K.L., Mashiyama, S.T., Morgan, M.A. et al. (1998). The Healthy Neighborhoods Project: A local health department's role in catalyzing community development. *Health Education and Behavior, 25*(2), 146-159.

Erikson, E. (1963). *Childhood and society.* New York: W.W. Norton.

Futterman, D., Chabon, B., & Hoffman, N.D. (2000). HIV and AIDS in adolescents. *Pediatric Clinics of North America, 47*(1), 171-188.

Green, L.W., George, M.A., Daniel, M., Frankish, C.J., Herbert, C.P., Bowie, W. et al. (1995). *Study of participatory research in health promotion.* Ottawa: Royal Society of Canada.

Israel, B.A., Schulz, A.J., Parker, E.A., & Becker, A.B. (1998). Review of community-based research: Assessing partnership approaches to improve public health. *Annual Review of Public Health, 19,* 173-202.

Kirby, D. (2001). Understanding what works and what doesn't in reducing adolescent sexual risk-taking. *Family Planning Perspectives, 33*(6), 276-281.

McKnight, J., & Kretzmann, J. (1990). *Mapping community capacity.* Evanston, IL: Center for Urban Affairs and Policy Research, Northwestern University.

Minkler, M. (2000). Participatory action research and healthy communities. *Public Health Reports, 115*(1&2), 191-197.

Minkler, M. (2004). *Community organizing and community building for health* (2nd ed.). New Brunswick, NJ: Rutgers University Press.

Reason, P. (1994). *Participation in human inquiry.* London: Sage.

Resnick, M.D., Bearman, P.S., Blum, R.W., Bauman, K.E., Harris, K.M., Jones, J. et al. (1997). Protecting adolescents from harm: Findings from the National Longitudinal Study on Adolescent Health. *Journal of the American Medical Association, 278*(10), 823-832.

Saleeby, D. (Ed.). (1997). *The strengths perspective in social work practice* (2nd ed.). NY: Longman.

Sanders-Phillips, K. (1996). The ecology of urban violence: Its relationship to health promotion behaviors in Black and Latino communities. *American Journal of Health Promotion, 10,* 308-317.

School Accountability Report Card School Year 2000-2001. Retrieved 7/7/2003, from http:www.wccusd.k12.ca.us/sarc/CDE_richmond_h.htm

Shaffer, R. (1983). *Beyond the dispensary.* Nairobi, Kenya: Amref.

Skogan, W.G. (1990). *Disorder and decline: Crime and the spiral of decay in American neighborhoods.* Berkeley, CA: University of California Press.

Spears, L. (1999, April 11). Picturing concerns: The idea is to take the messages to policy makers and to produce change. *Contra Costa Times,* pp. A27, A32.

State of California Master Birth File 1991-1999. *CHAPE Birth Easy file.* CCC data prepared by Brigid Simms, Contra Costa Health Services' Community Health Assessment, Planning, and Evaluation Group: 4/10/02.

Stoecker, R. (1999). Are academics irrelevant? *American Behavioral Scientist, 42*(5), 840-854.

Strack, R., & Magill, C. (2004). Engaging youth through photovoice. *Journal of Health Promotion Practice, 5*(1), 49-58.

Tencati, E., Kole, S.L., Feigher, E., Winkleby, M., & Altman, D.G. (2002). Teens as advocates for substance use prevention: Strategies for implementation. *Health Promotion Practice, 3*(1), 18-29.

Walker, W., Brunner, W., Wise, F., & Leivermann, C. (2003). *HIV/AIDS epidemiology report*. Contra Costa Health Services, Public Health Division, Communicable Diseases Programs.

Wallerstein, N. (1992). Powerlessness, empowerment, and health: Implications for health promotion programs. *American Journal of Health Promotion, 6*, 197-205.

Wallerstein, N. (2002). Empowerment to reduce health disparities. *Scandinavian Journal of Public Health, 30*(Supp 59), 72-77.

Wallerstein, N., Larson-Bright, M., Adams, A. R., & Rael, R. M. (2000, November 14). *Youth Link: A youth policy leadership program in New Mexico*. Paper presented at the American Public Health Association, Boston, MA.

Wallerstein, N., Sanchez-Merki, V., & Dow, L. (2005). Freirian praxis in health education and community organizing: A case study of an adolescent prevention program. In M. Minkler (Ed.), *Community organizing and community building for health* (2nd ed.). New Brunswick, NJ: Rutgers University Press.

Wang, C.C. (2003). Using photovoice as a participatory assessment and issue selection tool: A case study with the homeless in Ann Arbor. In M. Minkler & N. Wallerstein (Eds.), *Community-based participatory research for health* (pp. 176-196). San Francisco: Jossey-Bass.

Wang, C.C., & Burris, M. (1994). Empowerment through photo novella: Portraits of participation. *Health Education Quarterly, 21*, 171-186.

Wang, C.C., Yi, W., Tao, Z., & Carovano, K. (1998). Photovoice as a participatory health promotion strategy. *Health Promotion International, 13*(1), 75-86.

Watson, M. (2003). *Learning to trust: Transforming difficult elementary classrooms through developmental discipline*. San Francisco: Jossey-Bass.

Whaley, A.L. (1999). Preventing the high-risk sexual behavior of adolescents: Focus on HIV/AIDS transmission, unintended pregnancy, or both? *Journal of Adolescent Health, 24*(6), 376-382.

Wilson, N., Battistich, V., Syme, S.L., & Boyce, W.T. (2002). Does elementary school alcohol, tobacco and marijuana use increase middle school risk? *Journal of Adolescent Health, 30*(6), 442-447.

Wilson, N., Minkler, M., Dasho, S., Carrillo, R., Wallerstein, N., & Garcia, D. (2003). *Training students as partners in community based participatory prevention research: The Youth Empowerment Strategies (YES!) Project*. (Unpublished manuscript)

Wilson, N., Syme, S.L, Boyce, W.T., Battistich, V.A., & Selvin, S. (2005). Adolescent alcohol, tobacco, and marijuana use: The influence of neighborhood disorder and hope. *American Journal of Health Promotion, 20*(1), 11-19.

Wilson, W.J. (1996). *When work disappears: The world of the new urban poor*. NY: Alfred A. Knopf, Inc.

Yosihama, M., & Carr, E. S. (2002). Community participation reconsidered: Feminist participatory action research with Hmong women. *Journal of Community Practice, 10*(4), 85-103.

Zimmerman, M. A. (2000). Empowerment theory: Psychological, organizational and community levels of analysis. In J. Rappaport & E. Seidman (Eds.), *Handbook of community psychology* (pp. 43-63). NY: Academic/Plenum.

# Collaborative Teams for Youth Engagement

Julie A. Scheve, MEd
Daniel F. Perkins, PhD
Claudia Mincemoyer, PhD

**SUMMARY.** Youth engagement on collaborative teams is a viable approach to healthier youth development and community development. This article examines four characteristics of engagement in the research literature and a specific school-community-university project: adult support, a youth-friendly environment, the completion of meaningful tasks, and the learning and utilization of new skills. *[Article copies available for a fee from The Haworth Document Delivery Service: 1-800-HAWORTH. E-mail address: <docdelivery@haworthpress.com> Website: <http://www.HaworthPress. com> © 2006 by The Haworth Press, Inc. All rights reserved.]*

Julie A. Scheve, Daniel F. Perkins, and Claudia Mincemoyer are affiliated with the Department of Agricultural and Extension, The Pennsylvania State University.

Address correspondence to: Daniel F. Perkins, PhD, Associate Professor of Family and Youth Resiliency and Policy, The Pennsylvania State University, Department of Agricultural and Extension Education, 323 Agricultural Administration Building, University Park, PA 16802 (E-mail: dfp102@psu.edu).

The authors wish to acknowledge Ryan Stark, Assistant Professor of English, The Pennsylvania State University, and Amy Bertelsen, graduate student, Department of Agricultural and Extension Education, The Pennsylvania State University, for their comments on earlier drafts of this article.

The authors also wish to acknowledge the support of National Institute of Drug Abuse (1 R01 DA13709-01A1), Penn State University's Agricultural Experiment Station and Cooperative Extension Service.

[Haworth co-indexing entry note]: "Collaborative Teams for Youth Engagement." Scheve. Julie A., Daniel F. Perkins, and Claudia Mincemoyer. Co-published simultaneously in *Journal of Community Practice* (The Haworth Press, Inc.) Vol. 14, No. 1/2, 2006, pp. 219-234; and: *Youth Participation and Community Change* (ed: Barry N. Checkoway, and Lorraine M. Gutiérrez) The Haworth Press, Inc., 2006, pp. 219-234. Single or multiple copies of this article are available for a fee from The Haworth Document Delivery Service [1-800-HAWORTH, 9:00 a.m. - 5:00 p.m. (EST). E-mail address: docdelivery@haworthpress.com].

**KEYWORDS.** Youth engagement, youth development, prevention, collaboration, qualitative research

Opportunities for young people to engage in their communities have transcended community service and service-learning activities to include membership roles on school boards, city councils, boards of directors, and other positions of power. A growing amount of research captures the impact young people have when provided meaningful opportunities to contribute (Finn & Checkoway, 1998; Irby, Ferber, Pittman, Tolman, & Yohalem, 2001; Zeldin, 2004). With their energy, young people can reinvigorate adults and organizations by approaching challenges with a fresh perspective and offering creative solutions (Zeldin, McDaniel, Topitzes, & Calvert, 2000).

Youth service organizations may utilize youth engagement efforts to improve programs and services. Other traditional adult-held domains, such as collaborative teams, are beginning to recognize the advantages of including young people and are attempting to integrate them into their organizational operations and culture (Cargo, Grams, Ottoson, Ward, & Green, 2003; Checkoway, 1998; Hohenemser & Marshall, 2002). With the increasing interest of youth engagement on collaborative teams, a need exists to understand the ways in which collaborative teams can support youth engagement. This preliminary investigation examines youth engagement on collaborative teams focused on substance use prevention programming for middle school youth and their families. Currently, a dearth amount of research literature exists that explores youth involvement on collaborative teams focused on prevention services and programming (e.g., Einspruch & Wunrow, 2002).

The community teams are associated with the PROSPER (*PRO*moting *S*chool-community-university *P*artnerships to *E*nhance *R*esilience) partnership model (for a more detailed description see Spoth, Greenberg, Bierman, & Redmond, 2004). PROSPER links three existing national infrastructures to provide substance use prevention services to youth and families–the land-grant universities, the Cooperative Extension (CE) System, and the public school system. The partnership focuses on building community capacity to address public health issues. PROSPER teams exist in 14 rural communities in Pennsylvania and Iowa. Team membership includes CE educators, public school personnel, clergy, political leaders, law enforcement agents, parents, representatives from human service agencies (e.g., mental health professionals), and youth members. Approximately 10 adults and two high school youth comprise each team,

which meets at least monthly to coordinate and implement evidenced-based prevention programs.

Specifically, this preliminary study examines the ways in which adult
members support youth members' engagement efforts, how youth
members contribute to local teams, and what youth members learn
through their involvement on local teams. The following research questions guided the preliminary study: (a) In what ways do PROSPER
teams support youth engagement? (b) How do youth members contribute to their PROSPER teams? (c) What do youth members learn from
their experience on the PROSPER teams? and (d) Are engaged youth
members more likely to continue their participation on PROSPER
teams compared to youth members who are not engaged?

## LITERATURE REVIEW

Youth engagement efforts on collaborative teams embody the community youth development (CYD) framework. As an outgrowth of positive youth development in which young people are viewed as
resources, CYD views youth as partners in social change (Camino &
Zeldin, 2002) who can and should contribute to families, schools, organizations, and communities. Reviewing the current literature of youth
engagement on collaborative teams reveals four salient team characteristics that facilitate successful youth engagement efforts: adult support;
a youth-friendly environment; opportunities to complete meaningful
tasks; and opportunities to learn and use new skills (for a more
comprehensive review of these team characteristics see Scheve, 2005).

### Adult Support

A strong adult advocate of youth engagement may create an awareness of the need to include youth and foster consensus among the group
(Checkoway et al., 2003). Adults demonstrate support of youth engagement in a variety of ways. First, supportive adults display respect and
equality when working *with* youth (Camino, 2000). Second, supportive
adults clearly state expectations, responsibilities, and the time commitment required for youth to be engaged (Fiscus, 2003). Third, supportive
adults inform parents of their child's responsibilities as a member of the
team and make themselves available when parents have questions (Bernard, 2004). Fourth, supportive adults encourage youth to participate
during meetings by seeking their opinions or suggestions (Mueller,

Wunrow, & Einspruch, 2001). Finally, supportive adults regularly set aside time to reflect with youth (Kahne, Honig, & Mclaughlin, 1998). To ensure that youth members receive these types of support it may be necessary to establish an adult mentor for each youth member (Fiscus, 2003).

### Youth-Friendly Environment

To create an environment of inclusion where youth feel welcomed and appreciated, structural barriers which may prevent youth from participating need to be acknowledged and removed. Common barriers include lack of transportation to and from meetings, inconvenient meeting times and locations, and by-laws that restrict youth voting privileges (Young & Sazama, 1999). In addition to eliminating structural barriers, clear and ongoing communication between adults and youth is necessary. Mueller and colleagues (2000) recommend inviting youth to speak first at meetings to avoid feelings of intimidation that may discourage youth from participating as the meetings progress. However, allowing for youth input is not enough. Without listening to and *acting* on youth members' suggestions, youth engagement efforts may be weakened. Conversely, when youth feel their opinions are valued by the group, they are more likely to stay committed and involved (Fiscus, 2003).

### Opportunities to Complete Meaningful Tasks

Youth engagement efforts risk being devalued to tokenism, decoration, or even manipulation unless genuine opportunities exist for youth to participate in decision-making processes and complete meaningful tasks (Hart, 1992). In their work with youth-adult partnerships, Mueller and colleagues (2000) found that youth are more likely to remain engaged on collaborative teams when given increasing amounts of developmentally appropriate responsibilities. Therefore, the tasks youth perform should help the team meet overall goals and objectives. This type of experience may build civic competency, social connectedness, and social responsibility among youth (Checkoway et al., 2003). After the completion of projects, adults should engage youth in a reflection process to analyze what went well and what could be improved upon in the future (Huebner, 1998). Unexpected or disappointing outcomes should be planned for so that they become teachable moments in which youth learn how to take risks and "fail courageously" (Perkins & Borden, 2003, p. 334).

## Opportunities to Learn and Use New Skills

The CYD framework encourages opportunities for youth to learn new skills and experience a sense of mastery and self-efficacy (Perkins et al., 2003). Cargo and colleagues (2003) found that youth involved in a community health intervention experienced compromise, teamwork, cooperation, perspective-taking, and a breakdown of stereotypes through their involvement with the project. Such opportunities not only allow youth to build cognitive and social competencies (Listen, Inc., 2003) that can be applied to other areas of their life, but also may foster the development of initiative that often times is absent in school settings (Larson, 2000).

## METHODS

Researchers collected information by conducting structured telephone interviews with youth members on PROSPER teams. Interview questions were predetermined and asked in the same order to all participants (Denzin & Lincoln, 2000). The goal of the study was to understand youth members' experiences on the team by obtaining rich descriptions of their context and setting, thus, providing the rationale for open-ended, structured interviews (Marshall & Rossman, 1995). During the first phase of the interviews, permission to participate in the study was obtained from a parent and the youth member by telephone. Then, a time and date to complete the interview was scheduled with the youth member. During the second phase of the interviews, youth members were called at the predetermined time and the telephone interviews were completed on average within 24 minutes. The interviews were conducted by a graduate assistant affiliated with the PROSPER project. Participants were assured anonymity and told they could stop the interview at any time.

Twenty-four out of 36 current and previous youth members participated in structured telephone interviews (67% response rate). This method of purposeful sampling provided "information-rich cases" on the topics pertinent to the study (Patton, 1990). Youth members not interviewed were either unable to be reached by phone, unavailable at the scheduled interview time, or refused to participate in the study. Study participants ranged in age from 14-19, 63% were female and 94% were White. Fifteen participants resided in Pennsylvania and nine resided in Iowa.

Upon completion of the telephone interviews, youth members received copies of the questions and their answers to review and make elaborations or corrections (see Table 1 for a sample of the interview questions). This type of member check increases the credibility of the study (Erlandson, Harris, Skipper, & Allen, 1993). Seven of the twenty-four youth members interviewed had corrections or elaborations to their responses (29%).

## RESULTS

During the data analysis phase of the study, individual interview responses were segregated into independent ideas, which were written on note cards. Then, the note cards were sorted into categories that

TABLE 1. Sample of Youth Engagement Survey (YES) Interview Questions by Categories

Adult Support–3 questions total

1. Do you feel your opinions are respected by adults?* In what ways do adult members show/not show their respect for youth members?
2. If you miss a meeting does an adult member talk with you afterwards to keep you informed of what is happening on the team?
3. Does an adult member talk with you before or after meetings to reflect on the meetings?

Youth-Friendly Environment–3 questions total

1. Do you feel that adult members listen to your ideas and suggestions during the PROSPER team meetings?*
2. Do you feel that adult members act on your ideas and suggestions during the PROSPER team meetings?*

Opportunities to Complete Meaningful Tasks–3 questions total

1. As a youth member, what type of tasks do you perform?
2. Using a scale of 1 to 5 where 1 means not at all important and 5 means very important, overall how important are the tasks you perform to the team's goals?
3. Do adults assist you in the completion of tasks, projects, or ideas which you have?*

Opportunities to Learn and Use New Skills–2 questions total

1. What is the most important thing you have learned through your experience with the PROSPER team?
2. In what ways have you used the skills you've learned through your involvement with the PROSPER team in other areas of your life?

Closing

1. Imagine a scale from 1 to 5 where 1 is not at all connected and 5 is very connected. How connected do you feel to the PROSPER team?
2. Do you plan to stay involved with the PROSPER team next year? Why or why not? OR What were the reasons you did not stay involved with the PROSPER team?

Note. Questions with an * were used to gauge level of youth engagement on collaborative team (see Table 3).

emerged from the data (Erlandson et al., 1993). Finally, the categories were used to describe youth members' experiences of engagement.

### Adult Support

Adults display support of youth engagement efforts through their actions. Specifically, this category sought to understand if adults (a) respected the opinions of youth members, (b) reflected with youth members about meetings, and (c) contacted youth members if they missed a meeting.

Twenty-two youth (92%) felt adults respected their opinions during team meetings (see Table 2). Adults demonstrated respect by being attentive to youth members' ideas. One youth stated, "You could tell by their body language and nonverbal behavior that they [adults] were always paying attention to me and verbal cues that they were listening to me" (youth 124). Conversely, two youth (8%) did not feel respected by adults because they did not have opportunities to participate in discussions, an indicator of low engagement. One youth stated, "I wasn't really approached [by adults] for my opinions very much in the program" (youth 122).

Twelve youth (50%) stated that they participated in some form of a reflection process regarding the meetings. Meeting reflection occurred in two ways for youth members, either privately with an adult member or with the team at the beginning or end of the meeting. Fifteen youth (63%) stated they were contacted through email or postal mail when they missed a meeting.

### Youth-Friendly Environment

A youth-friendly environment shows that adults are intent on including youth in the organizational operations and culture. Specifically, this category examined if (a) meeting times were scheduled at a time when youth members could attend and (b) adults listened to and acted on youth members' ideas.

Five of the fourteen teams scheduled their monthly meetings in the after-school hours, making it possible for youth members to attend. Five teams scheduled their meetings during the school day and four teams had meeting times that varied from month to month. Such meeting times may pose challenges for youth members if they cannot be excused from school. Of the nine teams with meetings either during the school day or at various times throughout the day, four had made arrangements

TABLE 2. Youth Member Responses to the Youth Engagement Survey (YES) Interview Questions

| Questions | Yes | Sometimes | No | Total |
|---|---|---|---|---|
| **Adult Support** | | | | |
| Do you feel that your opinions are respected by adults? | 91.7% (22) | --- | 8.3% (2) | 100.0% (24) |
| Does an adult member talk with you before or after meeting to reflect on meetings? | 50.0% (12) | 8.3% (2) | 33.3% (8) | 91.6% (22)[a] |
| If you miss a meeting, does an adult member talk with you afterwards to keep you informed of what is happening on the team? | 62.5% (15) | 4.2% (1) | 20.8% (5) | 87.5% (21)[a, b] |
| **Youth-Friendly Environment** | | | | |
| Do you feel that adults listen to your ideas and suggestions during the PROSPER team meetings? | 91.7% (22) | --- | --- | 91.7% (22)[a] |
| Do you feel adult members act on your ideas and suggestions during the PROSPER team meetings? | 69.6% (16) | 8.7% (2) | 8.7% (2) | 87.0% (20)[a, c, d] |
| **Opportunities to Complete Meaningful Tasks** | | | | |
| Do adults assist you in the completion of tasks, projects, or ideas which you have? | 83.3% (20) | 4.2% (1) | 12.5% (3) | 100.0% (24) |
| **Opportunities to Learn and Use New Skills** | | | | |
| Have you learned something through your experience with the PROSPER team? | 100.0% (24) | --- | --- | 100.0% (24) |
| Have you used the skills you've learned through your experience with the PROPSER team in other areas of your life? | 87.0% (20) | --- | 13.0% (3) | 100.0% (23)[d] |

[a]Two youth members reported they did not attend PROSPER team meetings and therefore the question did not apply to them.

[b]One youth member reported that he has not missed a PROSPER team meeting and therefore the question did not apply to him.

[c]One youth member reported she did not know if adults acted on her ideas.

[d]For this question there is missing data for one youth member.

with school personnel to excuse youth members from class to attend team meetings.

Twenty-two youth (92%) stated that adults listened to their ideas during the team meetings (see Table 2). Two youth (8%) did not attend team meetings, thus they did not have a chance to voice their ideas, an indicator of low engagement. Fewer youth, sixteen (69%), stated that adults acted on their ideas while two youth (9%) reported adults sometimes acted on their ideas. Conversely, one youth (4%) did not know if adults acted on her ideas, two youth (9%) stated that adults did not act on their ideas, and two youth (9%) did not attend meetings: all indicators of low engagement. One youth interviewed did not answer this question. Youth members described adults acting on their ideas regarding the PROSPER prevention curriculum entitled *Strengthening Families Program 10-14* (SFP), which is offered to parents and their 6th grade children. One youth stated,

> We were all talking about what program to pick in our school. The adults were set on one and all of the youth [members] were like we are not sure that one is the best one for the youth [middle school students]. And we told them what plan we wanted to pick and we ended up doing that program because they respected our opinions and took our suggestion seriously. (youth 112)

## Opportunities to Complete Meaningful Tasks

Youth engagement on community collaboratives are sustained over time when adults create opportunities for youth to complete tasks which advance team goals. Specifically, this category sought examples of (a) tasks performed by youth members and (b) adults assisting youth members in the completion of tasks.

Eighteen (75%) youth stated they helped with the Strengthening Families Program 10-14. Tasks included: recruiting 6th grade students into the program, helping with child care during program sessions, participating on a youth panel, coordinating program meals, taking pictures, and co-facilitating the youth portion of program sessions. The second most frequent task performed by youth members was providing ideas at meetings (63%) followed by recruiting other youth to join the team (13%). Most youth (83%) reported completing more than one task.

Youth members were asked to rate the level of importance their tasks were to achieving their team's overall goals using a Likert-type scale with 1 = least important to 5 = most important. Of the twenty-four youth, sixteen (67%) stated their tasks were very important to achieving teams' goals, five youth (21%) stated their tasks were somewhat important to achieving teams' goals, and three youth (12%) stated their tasks were not at all important to achieving teams' goals. The mean score for youth perception's of the level of importance their tasks were to achieving overall team goals was 3.4. In addition, as the perception levels of tasks' importance increased among youth members, so did their feelings of connectedness to their teams ($r = .596$, df = 22, $p < .002$).

To complete tasks, twenty youth members (83%) stated they received assistance from adults while one youth (4%) stated she sometimes received assistance from adults (see Table 3). Conversely, three youth (13%) stated they did not receive assistance from adults when completing tasks, an indicator of low engagement. Two youth described the kind of assistance they received in their responses below.

> When we did a skit to recruit 6th graders during school time, one of the members worked in the same school building that we [youth members] were at and she helped with some of the planning of the skit. (youth 104)

> Every night at the PROSPER sessions, when I was an arranger, all of the facilitators would help me with the meals. Especially on the first night [the team leader] helped me figure things out and explained to me what my job was. It made me feel more comfortable because I was nervous before I went. (youth 116)

## Opportunities to Learn and Use New Skills

Youth participation in meaningful tasks that advance team goals creates opportunities for youth to learn new skills. As a result, they may apply the new skills into other areas of their lives. Specifically, this category sought examples of (a) new skills learned by youth and (b) how youth applied the skills in other areas of their lives.

TABLE 3. Cross Tabulation of Youth Engagement and Team Connection

| Level of youth engagement | Low team connection | | High team connection | |
|---|---|---|---|---|
| | Number of participants | Percent | Number of participants | Percent |
| High: No negative response to the four categories | 5 | 29.4 | 12 | 70.6 |
| Medium: 1 negative response to the four categories | 1 | 33.3 | 2 | 66.7 |
| Low: 2-4 negative responses to the four categories | 3 | 100.0 | 0 | 0 |

$\chi^2 = 5.38$, df = 2, p < .068

Note. The selected questions to gauge level of youth engagement asked whether youth felt adults respected them, assisted them, listened to their ideas, and acted on their ideas. One youth interviewed did not answer one of the four selected levels of youth engagement questions.

Seventeen youth (71%) described learning life skills such as teamwork, responsibility, and commitment (see Table 2). Other responses included a greater understanding of how PROSPER helps people (38%), how youth can play a role on the team (13%), how youth can help in their communities (13%), how to organize an event (8%), and how to be a positive role model to younger kids (8%). Most youth (79%) reported learning more than one skill. One youth stated, "Most important was working with a group that had a diverse background–adults, youth, people with different ethnic backgrounds, people from all parts of the community. And it helped me to work with diverse groups of people" (youth 119).

Twenty-one (87%) youth found ways to apply the skills they learned through PROSPER in other areas of their lives. Youth described feeling more comfortable working in a team environment (44%), and having a greater awareness of their relationship with others in their lives (26%). One youth stated, "I'm in college now so it's been a benefit because it is easier to work with groups and work on class projects and be able to get along with more people" (youth 119). "With PROSPER, it is like you learn to care and devote time to other people–other than your friends, boyfriends, or family. It is outside of your normal bubble" (youth 115).

Other responses included being more responsible about commitments (13%), being more comfortable talking with kids or adults (17%), being more ambitious (4%), being a better student (4%), and being able to organize church events (4%). Many youth reported using more than one skill in other areas of their lives. Three youth (13%) felt they did not use skills learned through their involvement with PROSPER in other areas of their lives. One youth interviewed did not answer this question.

In wrapping up the interview, youth were asked if they planned to stay involved with their team or why they were no longer involved with the team. Twenty youth (84%) wanted to stay involved with their team or remained with their team until they moved away to attend college and two youth (8%) discontinued their involvement due to their commitment to sports.

Two youth (8%) were unsure about remaining involved with their team because they felt little current involvement. One youth stated, "I don't know. I'm not doing anything now. I'm not involved now" (youth 102). Each of these participants also rated their level of task importance and connection to the team as a 2 or lower on a 5 point Likert-type scale with higher answers indicating high importance and connection.

Four questions were closely examined to gain a sense of youth's level of engagement. The selected questions asked whether youth felt adults respected them, assisted them, listened to their ideas, and acted on their ideas. Levels of engagement were grouped into three different categories: (a) No negative responses to any of the four questions (in other words these participants said yes to the four questions); (b) one negative response to any of the four questions; and (c) 2-4 negative responses. Next, a cross-tabulation comparison was run to explore possible differences of level of engagement on team connectedness (measured by a Likert-type scale with 1 = not at all connected to 5 = very connected; see Table 3). Participants' team connectedness responses were separated into two categories, low (1-3.4) and high (3.5-5).

Twenty-nine percent of participants with no negative engagement responses felt a low connection to the team; this increased to 33% and 100% of participants with 1 negative response and 2-4 negative responses, respectively. One youth interviewed did not answer 1 of the 4 selected levels of youth engagement questions. The Chi square test for differences among the groups approached significance ($\chi^2 = 5.38$, df = 2, p < .068); however, the cell sizes were small. A possible threshold exists; that is, more than one negative experience is needed before youth feel disconnected from the team. Feeling disconnected may lead youth to not stay involved with the team.

## DISCUSSION

This study examined youth engagement on collaborative teams affiliated with PROSPER. Researchers sought to understand the experiences of PROSPER youth members through structured telephone interviews. Youth members were asked about the presence of team characteristics found in the literature to facilitate successful youth engagement.

Youth engagement on collaborative teams begins with adult support. Findings from this study show that adult members demonstrated support of youth members mostly by respecting their opinions. Less common was for adults to reflect with youth regarding meetings or to contact youth when they missed a meeting. Reflecting with youth members about meeting discussions and providing information to them when they miss a meeting ensures that youth members have the information they need to offer an opinion. Thus, practitioners who engage youth on collaborative teams may want to designate an adult member as a mentor, who can set aside time to reflect with youth on meeting discussions and follow-up with youth members when they miss a meeting.

A youth-friendly environment fosters youth engagement on collaborative teams. Findings from this study show that adults may not always schedule team meetings at convenient times. In this study, 65% of the teams scheduled meetings during school hours or their meeting times varied. If youth members cannot attend team meetings, then their ability to voice opinions and contribute to discussions is limited. Thus, practitioners who want to increase youth's engagement on collaborative teams may want to consider convenience of their meeting times and request that school personnel excuse youth members from class to attend team meetings when necessary.

Opportunities for youth members to complete meaningful tasks may sustain youth engagement efforts over time. Findings from this study show that a majority of youth members completed meaningful tasks and also appreciated the assistance they received from adults in the process. Completing meaningful tasks may bring a sense of purpose to the role of youth members. Moreover, when adults assist youth members in the completion of tasks, it may prevent youth members from feeling nervous or overwhelmed. Thus, practitioners who want to engage youth on collaborative teams may want to identify specific tasks for youth that advance overall goals and also have adult mentors assist youth members in the completion of these tasks.

Youth engagement on collaborative teams creates opportunities for youth members to learn skills outside of traditional classroom settings. Findings from this study show that a majority of youth members learned skills which they applied to their school work and interpersonal relationships. Thus, practitioners who want to continue youth engagement efforts on collaborative teams may want to schedule time with each youth member (e.g., an informal meeting at an ice cream shop) to reflect on the tasks the youth member has completed and the skills he or she has learned.

The present study provides initial insight on four team characteristics found in the literature that promote youth engagement on collaborative teams–adult support, a youth-friendly environment, opportunities to complete meaningful tasks, and opportunities to learn and use new skills. Three limitations exist in this study. First, interview participants may have provided socially desirable answers; however, to reduce this likelihood, participants were ensured anonymity. Second, youth members were the source for all of the data collected in the study. This study would have been enhanced by utilizing data triangulation (Denzin, 1978, as cited in Patton, 1990), which would have included interviews from PROSPER team leaders and adult members. Finally, structured interviews set limits on topics discussed during the interviews. Semi-structured interviews would have allowed youth to discuss issues that were important to them and unknown to researchers.

Future research may want to examine the effectiveness of such team efforts in addressing community issue as compared to adult-only community teams. Future research may also examine the team characteristics that most influence the retention of youth members and the environmental factors (e.g., neighborhood organization, team readiness, and poverty) that may influence the relationship between youth and adult members. Moreover, longitudinal research is needed to examine youth experiences over time, and whether the negative experiences influence continued involvement.

In summary, youth engagement on collaborative teams may create opportunities for youth to build competencies, connect with non-familial adults, and impact change within their communities. Collaborative teams may benefit from youth participation in terms of youth's enthusiasm, fresh ideas, and closeness to the youth audience. In a time when youth are increasingly isolated from adults and absent from our society's political conversations, the community youth development framework, which promotes youth engagement on collaborative teams, provides practitioners with a guide to reconnect youth to their communities.

# REFERENCES

Bernard, H. (2004). The power of an untapped resource: Exploring youth representation on your board or committee. Juneau, AK: The Association of Alaska School Boards. Retrieved from website on March 15, 2004, *http://www.aasb.org/Publications. html*.

Camino, L. (2000). Youth-adult partnerships: New territory in community work and research. *Applied Developmental Science, 4,* 11-20.

Camino, L., & Zeldin, S. (2002). Making the transition to community youth development: Emerging roles and competencies for youth-serving organizations and youth workers. *Community Youth Development Journal,* 70-78.

Cargo, M., Grams, G., Ottoson, J., Ward, P., & Green, L. (2003). Empowerment as fostering positive youth development and citizenship. *Journal of Health Behavior, 27,* S66-S79.

Checkoway, B. (1998). Involving young people in neighborhood development. *Children and Youth Services Review, 20,* 765-795.

Checkoway, B., Richards-Schuster, K., Abdullah, S., Aragon, M., Facio, E., Figueroa, L., Reddy, E., Welsh, M., & White, A. (2003). Young people as competent citizens. *Community Development Journal, 28,* 298-309.

Denzin, N. K. (1978). *The research act: A theoretical introduction to sociological methods.* New York: McGraw-Hill.

Denzin, N. K., & Lincoln, Y. S. (2000). *Handbook of qualitative research* (2nd ed.). Thousand Oaks, CA: Sage Publications.

Einspruch, E., & Wunrow, J. J. (2002). Assessing youth/adult partnerships: The seven circles (AK) experience. *Journal of Drug Education, 32*, 1-12.

Erlandson, D. A., Harris, E. L., Skipper, B. L., & Allen, S. D. (1993). *Doing Naturalistic Inquiry*. Newbury Park, CA: Sage Publications.

Finn, J. L., & Checkoway, B. (1998). Young people as competent community builders: A challenge to social work. *Social Work, 43*, 335-345.

Fiscus, L. (2003). Youth as equal partners in decision making. *The Education Digest, 68*, 58-63.

Hart, R. (1992). *Children's participation: From tokenism to citizenship*. Florence, Italy: International Child Development Center, UNIEF.

Hohenemser, L., & Marshall, B. (2002). Utilizing a youth development framework to establish and maintain a youth advisory committee. *Health Promotion Practice, 3*, 155-165.

Huebner, A. J. (1998). Examining "empowerment": A how-to-guide for the youth development professional. *Journal of Extension*, 36. Retrieved from website on Jan. 22, 2004, *http://www.joe.org/joe/1998december/a1.html*.

Irby, M., Ferber, T., & Pittman, K., Tolman, J., Yohalem, N. (2001). *Youth action: Youth contributing to communities, communities supporting youth*. Takoma Park, MD: Forum for Youth Investment, International Youth Foundation.

Kahne, J., Honig, M., & Mclaughlin, M. W. (1998). The civic components of community youth development. *New Designs for Youth Development, 14*, 9-11.

Larson, R. (2000). Toward a psychology of positive youth development. *American Psychologist, 55*, 170-183.

Listen Inc., (2003). *An emerging model for working with youth: Community organizing + youth development = youth organizing*. New York City, New York: Funders' Collaborative on Youth Organizing. Retrieved from website on March 15, 2004, *http://www.fcyo.org/sitebody/resources.htm*.

Marshall, C., & Rossman, G. B. (1995). *Designing qualitative research*. Thousand Oaks, CA: Sage Publications.

Mueller R. B., Wunrow, J. J., & Einspruch, E. L. (2000). Providing youth services through youth-adult partnerships: A review of the literature. *Reaching Today's Youth, 4*, 37-48.

Patton, M. Q. (1990). *Qualitative evaluation and research methods* (2nd ed.). Newbury Park, CA: Sage Publications.

Perkins, D. F., & Borden, L. M. (2003). Key elements of community youth development. In Villarruel, F. A., Perkins, D. F., Borden, L. M., & Keith, J. G. (Eds.), *Community Youth Development: Programs, policies, and practices* (pp. 327-340). Thousand Oaks, CA: Sage Publications.

Perkins, D. F., Borden, L. M., Keith, J. G., Hoope-Rooney, T. L., & Villarruel, F. A. (2003). Community youth development: Partnership creating a positive world. In Villarruel, F. A., Perkins, D. F., Borden, L. M., & Keith, J. G. (Eds.), *Community Youth Development: Programs, policies, and practices* (pp. 1-24). Thousand Oaks, CA: Sage Publications.

Scheve, J. A., (2005). *Say Y.E.S. to youth: Youth engagement strategies.* Unpublished manuscript. University Park, PA: The Pennsylvania State University, Department of Agricultural and Extension Education.

Spoth, R., Greenberg, M., Bierman, K., & Redmond, C. (2004). PROSPER community-university partnership model for public education systems: Capacity-building for evidenced-based, competence-building prevention. *Prevention Science, 5,* 31-39.

Wunrow, J. J., & Einspruch, E. L. (2001). Promoting youth-adult partnerships: The seven circles coalition in Sitka, Alaska. *The Journal of Primary Prevention, 22,* 169-185.

Young, K. S., & Sazama, J. (1999). *14 Points: Successfully involving youth in decision making.* Somerville, MA: Youth on Board.

Zeldin, S., McDaniel, A. K., Topitzes, D., & Calvert, M. (2000). *Youth in decision-making: A study on the impacts of youth on adults and organizations.* Washington, DC: National 4-H Council.

Zeldin, S. (2004). Youth as agents of adult and community development: Mapping the processes and outcomes of youth engaged in organizational governance. *Applied Developmental Science, 8, 75-90.*

# OUTCOMES OF YOUTH ORGANIZING AND OTHER APPROACHES

## Youth Organizing, Identity-Support, and Youth Development Agencies as Avenues for Involvement

Michelle Alberti Gambone, PhD
Hanh Cao Yu, PhD
Heather Lewis-Charp, MA
Cynthia L. Sipe, PhD
Johanna Lacoe, BA

**SUMMARY.** What are the differences in outcomes among youth organizing and other efforts to involve young people at the community level?

Michelle Alberti Gambone is President, Youth Development Strategies, Inc., Philadelphia, PA. Hanh Cao Yu and Heather Lewis-Charp are affilated with Social Policy Research Associates, Oakland, CA. Cynthia L. Sipe works with Youth Development Strategies, Inc., Lansdale, PA. Johanna Lacoe lives and works in New York City.

Address all correspondence to: Michelle Alberti Gambone, PhD, President, Youth Development Strategies, Inc., 429 Fulton Street, Philadelphia, PA 19147 (E-mail: mgambone@ydsi.org).

This paper was made possible by the Center for Information and Research on Civic Learning and Engagement, the Ford Foundation, and the Innovation Center for Youth and Community Development.

[Haworth co-indexing entry note]: "Youth Organizing, Identity-Support, and Youth Development Agencies as Avenues for Involvement." Gambone, Michelle Alberti et al. Co-published simultaneously in *Journal of Community Practice* (The Haworth Press, Inc.) Vol. 14, No. 1/2, 2006, pp. 235-253; and: *Youth Participation and Community Change* (ed: Barry N. Checkoway, and Lorraine M. Gutiérrez) The Haworth Press, Inc., 2006, pp. 235-253. Single or multiple copies of this article are available for a fee from The Haworth Document Delivery Service [1-800-HAWORTH, 9:00 a.m. - 5:00 p.m. (EST). E-mail address: docdelivery@haworthpress.com].

This paper examines differences in developmental outcomes among youth organizing, identity-support, and traditional youth development agencies, with the finding that there are significant differences in outcomes such as civic activism and identity development. It reports that youth organizing agencies show higher levels of youth leadership, decision making, and community involvement in comparison with other agencies, and concludes that deliberate approaches to staffing and decision-making can influence youth outcomes. *[Article copies available for a fee from The Haworth Document Delivery Service: 1-800-HAWORTH. E-mail address: <docdelivery@haworthpress.com> Website: <http://www.HaworthPress.com>* © 2006 by The Haworth Press, Inc. All rights reserved.]

**KEYWORDS.** Youth development, civic activism, identity development, developmental outcomes, comparative analysis

## INTRODUCTION

A key tenet of youth's development is their ability to increasingly recognize their potential to making contributions to the public sphere. Yet, young people's knowledge of civic and political systems is generally superficial and not action-oriented (Torney-Purta, Lehmann, Oswald, & Schultz, 2001). In fact, civic education in public schools provides the kind of fact-based knowledge and teacher-driven learning experience that limits youth's direct engagement in real-world processes of decision making and political processes (Larson & Hansen, 2004).

Youth development organizations provide a logical setting for civic engagement because, as an approach, youth development is an inclusive strategy that strives to provide *the* key developmental "supports and opportunities" that young people need for healthy growth. While youth development models and approaches have always emphasized the importance of community involvement, the late 1990s saw leaders in the field advocating more applied forms of community engagement, such as youth-action or youth activism (Irby, Ferber & Pittman, 2001; Hughes & Curnan, 2002; Kahne, Honig, & McLaughlin, 2002; Sullivan, 1997).

Youth development agencies that are looking to provide applied civic engagement opportunities can draw on various models of youth activism for inspiration, including, most prominently, the work of youth organizing agencies. As of yet, however, there has been little research on whether youth activism approaches are developmentally appropriate and compatible with the youth development paradigm. In other words, there is little evidence that youth activism approaches are effective at achieving desired community engagement outcomes and/or at supporting the holistic development of youth (Sherrod, 2000; Michelsen, Zaff & Hair, 2002).

In an effort to address this gap in the youth development literature, this research uses a developmental "supports and opportunities" framework (Connell, Gambone, & Smith, 2000) to examine the work of two different types of youth activism organizations, namely "youth organizing" and "identity support" agencies. Two key research questions guided this work:

- Do youth in organizing and identity-support organizations experience developmental supports and opportunities at different levels than youth in more traditional youth development organizations?
- Are there differences in levels of key developmental outcomes between youth organizing, identity-support, and traditional youth development organizations?

### Analytical Typology

The differentiation, used throughout this article, between "youth organizing" and "identity-support" was arrived at inductively from a three-year qualitative study of nine youth activism organizations (Lewis-Charp, Yu, Soukamneuth, & Lacoe, 2003). Below we briefly provide a description of each "type," with a more complete summary of organizational and programmatic practices provided in Table 1.

Youth within organizing agencies honed their political participation and critical thinking skills by asserting their voices on key issues in their communities. *Youth organizing* approaches included political education, community mapping, public protest, letter-writing campaigns, and public awareness movements. Each agency consisted of "core youth organizers" or "youth staff," an unpaid "youth membership," and at least one young adult leader. Youth within these agencies tended to be racially and/or ethnically diverse. Youth organizing agencies described in this study have led successful campaigns to increase language access in standardized tests, lobbied against punitive California legislation that would lead to increased youth incarceration, organized against toxic waste facilities in their low-income communities, and sought to create new forms of community policing.

TABLE 1. Summary of Key Characteristics of Youth Organizing and Identity-Support Organizations

|  | Youth Organizing Practices | Identity-Support Practices |
|---|---|---|
| Organizational Level | • Youth work on staff and/or stipends paid for youth organizers<br>• Core youth "organizers" and broader youth "membership"<br>• Priority on grassroots empowerment and youth voice<br>• Diverse youth groups targeted<br>• Community change focus | • Use of adult volunteers (role models and support)<br>• Core youth "leaders" and broader group of youth who access services<br>• Priority on safe space<br>• Single identity groups targeted<br>• Individual development focus |
| Programmatic Level | • Celebration of youth culture and voice.<br>• Political education on social movements, political processes, current events<br>• Campaign development<br>• Direct action such as letter writing campaigns, petition drives, protest, and boycott | • Celebration of culture and racial, ethnic, and sexual identity.<br>• Critical education on history of ethnic, racial, or sexual identity group.<br>• Workshops on issues of power and oppression; support groups<br>• Community education and advocacy on identity-specific issues |

*Identity support* agencies fostered opportunities for marginalized young people from a specific ethnic, racial, or social group (e.g., African-American youth, gay and lesbian youth, etc.) to reflect on issues of personal and group identity, with an emphasis on building an autonomous yet socially integrated and connected sense of self. Identity support approaches included "critical" education about the history and politics of the identity group, interactive and experiential learning, support groups, and community outreach, education, and advocacy. Community engagement within these groups focused broadly on civic awareness and connectedness rather than organized social action. Identity support groups relied extensively on adult volunteers, using a youth-adult partnership model of leadership, and placed a very high priority on the creation and maintenance of safe space.

### About the Research Study

The findings reported in this article draw on data generated as part of an evaluation of the Youth Leadership Development Initiative (YLDI). The original data from the YLDI study came from a group of nine organizations that utilized one of two key programming strategies–identity support or youth organizing. Findings from the evaluation suggested that youth organizing and identity support programs show promise in addressing the alienation and disengagement of marginalized young people from civic life. Evidence suggests they present opportunities for political socialization different from other youth-serving institutions because they strive to respond to issues of relevance to youth and address basic issues of personal and social identity as an entrée to civic action (Lewis-Charp et al., 2003). Additionally, such organizations emphasize respect for diversity and put youth in roles as leaders–where young people, rather than adults, construct meanings and understandings of public spheres (Camino & Shepherd, 2002; Torney-Purtra, 1999). While much existing research documents youths' marginalization from civic participation and society because of their race, ethnicity, class, gender, sexual orientation, and immigrant status, the YLDI research focused attention on the ways that youth organizing and identity support enable young people to act upon their desire to change the forces that relegate them to the margins (Mohamed & Wheeler, 2001).

A limitation of the original YLDI study was its lack of reference to other types of youth programming against which youths' developmental experiences within this type of organization could be considered. In order to strengthen and expand our findings, we administered a youth survey to a comparison group of eight organizations. This article summarizes the results of this comparative analysis, identifies policy implications, and frames questions for further research on each of these strategies based on the quantitative data collected.

## METHODOLOGY

### Respondents

We administered a survey to *all* of the participating youth in nine of the YLDI organizations, including *four* identity support and *five* youth organizing. To get a comparative perspective of the effectiveness of different programmatic approaches, we recruited and selected eight predominately urban organizations for the "traditional" youth development programs, in five states that met the following criteria: (1) targeted older, diverse youth, and (2) had a programmatic focus that involved youth in their communities. The agencies included a Boys & Girls' club, conservation corps, a community garden project, arts organizations, and youth leadership organizations. These organizations were provided with a stipend for their participation in the study and a thorough orientation to ensure their understanding and proper administration of the survey instrument.

Table 2 provides a summary of the total number and characteristics of youth in the study groups; these groups are demographically very comparable. The mean age of all respondents was between 15 and 16 years old. However, the survey respondents from the youth organizing and comparison groups had been attending the organizations slightly longer and more frequently than those from the identity support groups. How representative are the participants of the population of youth involved in the three types of organizations? Within each organization *all* youth who participate were included in the survey (i.e., we surveyed the population rather than a sample–so that no inferences needed to be made to the participants of the programs in the study). However, we do not claim that our sample represents all youth activism programs. Only that as a exploratory research this work points us to important differences that warrant a larger scale, more systematic study of these issues.

## Survey Measures

The youth development framework of Connell, Gambone and Smith (2000) provides a road map that identifies desired long-term outcomes

TABLE 2. Demographic Profile of Survey Respondents

|  | I. Identity Support YLDI Agencies (N = 145) | II. Youth Organizing YLDI Agencies (N = 65) | III. Youth Development Comparison Agencies (N = 257) |
|---|---|---|---|
| **Race/Ethnicity** | | | |
| African American | 64% | 27% | 44% |
| Hispanic | 0% | 23% | 13% |
| White | 11% | 12% | 16% |
| Asian & Pacific Islander | 17% | 30% | 7% |
| Other/Multi-Racial | 9% | 8% | 18% |
| **Age** | | | |
| Mean age | 16.5 | 16.6 | 15.0 |
| **Time in Program** | | | |
| At org 3 Months or Less | 44% | 24% | 25% |
| At org > 1 yr | 44% | 60% | 60% |
| **Frequency of Attendance** | | | |
| Attend every day | 11% | 54% | 41% |

for young people and articulates the youth development practices needed to achieve these outcomes. Specifically, the framework focuses on the supports and opportunities that young people need to experience in order to attain key developmental outcomes (i.e., learning to be productive, to connect and to navigate) as they move toward long-term, early adult outcomes. Community strategies such as civic engagement programs are expected to enhance developmental outcomes through the provision of these supports and opportunities (see Figure 1).

In designing the research project, we operationalized each of the components in the theory of change relative to the work and goals of the organizations in the YLDI project. The developmental outcomes (Figure 1, Box B) measured are: (1) *Civic activism*, so that young people can participate in civic action with a sense of efficacy, and the capacity for community problem solving (11 items, alpha = .90); (2) *Identity development*, so that young people experience a sense of affirmation of their identity and the ability to explore the different aspects of their identity (12 items, alpha = .89); and (3) *Coping*, so that young people increase the number of positive, or healthy, coping strategies they use, and decrease the number of negative, or unhealthy, coping strategies they use (6 items, alpha = .51).

We also measured youth's experience of *supports and opportunities* (Figure 1, Box C) in five areas using YDSI's youth survey. *Supportive relationships* assess the extent to which young people experience guidance, emotional and practical support and whether adults and peers know them and what is important to them (10 items, alpha = .86). *Safety* assesses

FIGURE 1.

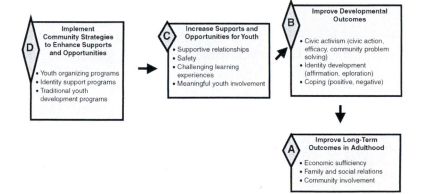

young people's experience of physical and emotional security (8 items, alpha = .51). *Youth involvement* assesses how young people are involved in meaningful roles with responsibility, that is, having input into decision-making, having opportunities for leadership, and feeling a sense of belonging (13 items, alpha = .87). *Skill building* assesses young people's experiences of challenging and interesting learning activities that help them build a wide array of skills, and experience a sense of growth and progress (7 items, alpha = .79). *Community involvement* measures young people's understanding of the greater community and having opportunities to give back to their community (6 items, alpha = .79).

According to supports and opportunities theory, participation in different experiences (e.g., in the case of this study, organizations' community-based activities) should contribute to general developmental growth (e.g., civic activism as political engagement of youth) for the young person. For this article, we are interested in beginning to explore how the different types of activities of these organizations relate to the levels of supports and opportunities youth receive and their levels of developmental growth in the three important developmental areas described above.

### Analysis Method

We used a non-traditional method to analyze the survey data that shows the results in terms of youth's experiences measured against a standard, rather than conventional ways of looking at mean levels. The standard is created by looking across the questions for each of the supports and opportunities (e.g., supportive relationships) and developmental outcomes (e.g., civic activism) to see whether the pattern of answers indicates that youth are consistently experiencing all of the relevant developmental dimensions of that area.

For example, in supportive relationships, if a youth's responses indicate they consistently have adults to go to for guidance, emotional support, practical support, etc., that youth's experience of supportive relationships is rated as developmentally optimal. Conversely, if a young person's responses indicate they consistently do not get these benefits from relationships with adults in the program, they are rated as having a developmentally insufficient experience. In this way we can see what proportion of the youth in a program are having experiences that reach the highest standard (i.e., optimal) and what proportion might be having experiences that do not meet the standard of being developmentally rich (i.e., insufficient).

We conducted chi square tests to determine whether there were significant differences in the proportion of youth who are having optimal or insufficient experiences and outcomes among the three groups: identity-focused, youth organizing and traditional youth development organizations. In addition, paired t-tests were used to determine whether there were significant differences between: (1) youth organizing and identity support agencies; (2) youth organizing and traditional agencies; and (3) identity support and traditional agencies.

## Qualitative Data

In discussing the survey results, we are able to draw on rich data from a qualitative study of the identity support and youth organizing agencies. As part of an evaluation study these data were collected during two rounds of three day site visits to the eleven identity support and youth organizing agencies, which included observations, extensive one-on-one and focus group interviews with program staff, youth participants, youth leaders, and community members. Youth participants were recruited based upon staff's nomination of those who represent different length of participation in the program. Since the comparison organizations ('traditional' youth development) were not part of the evaluation they were not included in the site visits. However, we have some program information on the mission goals, and activities of our comparison organizations.

## FINDINGS FROM THIS STUDY

In order to address our key questions we compared the results of the youth survey in two ways. First, we compared the organizing and identity development organizations with each other. Next, we compared those organizations to the traditional youth development agencies.

## Developmental Outcomes

Developmental theory and research has shown that achieving healthy outcomes as an adult requires that youth reach key developmental milestones during their adolescence. These milestones can be characterized as learning to be productive, learning to be connected, and learning to navigate (Gambone et al., 2002; Connell, Gambone, & Smith, 2000). We measured one outcome in each developmental area. It is important

to keep in mind that developmental outcomes represent accomplishments of youth that are affected by the sum of their experiences, over
time, in different settings. As such, these are outcomes that programs
can contribute to only in the limited time they have contact with participants. Programs have relatively less ability to single-handedly change
these outcomes than they do youth's experiences of supports and opportunities.

Table 3 shows the percentage of youth demonstrating optimal or insufficient levels of each of the developmental outcomes. Column I contains data
for the YLDI agencies classified as identity support programs; Column II
has data for the YLDI agencies classified as youth organizing programs;
and Column III shows data for the traditional youth development agencies.
We found significant differences across the three types of agencies in the
proportions of youth in two of the three outcome areas measured.

TABLE 3. Developmental Outcomes by Agency Type

| | I. Identity Support YLDI Agencies (145) | | II. Youth Organizing YLDI Agencies (65) | | III. General Youth Development Comparison Agencies (257) | | |
|---|---|---|---|---|---|---|---|
| | Insufficient | Optimal | Insufficient | Optimal | Insufficient | Optimal | |
| **Civic Activism Overall** | 34% | 33% | 18% | 42% | 52% | 20% | *** |
| Civic Action | 28% | 30% | 15% | 42% | 42% | 19% | *** |
| Efficacy/ Agency | 10% | 46% | 6% | 40% | 23% | 26% | *** |
| Community Problem Solving | 11% | 33% | 3% | 37% | 23% | 20% | *** |
| **Identity Develop- ment Overall** | 2% | 55% | 6% | 34% | 21% | 16% | *** |
| Affirmation | 1% | 62% | 3% | 46% | 20% | 21% | *** |
| Exploration | 12% | 42% | 14% | 31% | 38% | 12% | *** |
| **Coping Overall** | 12% | 67% | 14% | 63% | 18% | 58% | ns |
| Positive Coping | 10% | 54% | 9% | 49% | 21% | 49% | ns |
| Negative Coping | 15% | 59% | 15% | 55% | 15% | 53% | ns |

***Significant differences between groups at .001

*Civic Activism.* Higher proportions of youth in both identity support and youth organizing agencies report optimal levels on the indicators of this outcome–civic action, efficacy and community problem solving–compared with youth in the traditional youth development agencies. About 40 percent of youth in the *youth organizing* agencies are optimal on civic activism overall and on each of the indicators of civic activism. About one-third of youth in the *identity support* agencies are optimal on these indicators as well (with the exception of efficacy, where 46% of youth are in the optimal category). Although the proportions are somewhat higher on the indicators for youth in the youth organizing agencies than they are for youth in the identity support programs, the differences are not statistically significant. Both types of civic engagement agencies, however, have significantly higher proportions of youth demonstrating optimal levels of civic activism outcomes than do the traditional youth development agencies.

We know that many traditional youth development organizations provide only limited opportunities for youth to participate in community service types of activities. Where these opportunities do exist they usually occur only periodically and for small numbers of the most engaged youth. Even fewer youth seem to have opportunities in these programs to explore the communities around them and understand how they can play a role in their communities. Given the lack of emphasis on this area in programming, the findings here are consistent with our expectations that fewer youth in traditional settings have attained the civic activism outcomes measured in this study.

*Identity Development.* As we would anticipate, youth in identity support agencies fare better in terms of identity outcomes–identity affirmation and identity exploration–than either of the other type agencies. Although the identity support agencies were strongest of the three types in this area, the youth organizing agencies also have significantly more youth at optimal levels of these indicators than did the traditional youth development agencies.

Qualitative data indicate that identity development is linked to specific practices within YLDI agencies. Identity-support agencies celebrate and affirm the ethnic, racial, cultural, and/or sexual identity of youth participants. They provide information on the history, art, and spiritual traditions of youths' identity group, and work to equip youth with knowledge and skills to deal with prejudice. Key program strategies included support groups, consciousness raising (through critical self-reflection), and cultural celebrations. Youth organizing agencies had less of an explicit focus on identity, and yet they too overtly discussed issues of identity within the context of the community issues they were addressing.

*Coping.* Coping is the only developmental outcome for which all agencies look similar. There were no significant differences among these agencies on either indicator of coping skills–negative coping or positive coping. In fact, half to two-thirds of the youth participating in all of the agencies fall into the optimal range of the coping measure used in this study. Because we did not collect qualitative data on strategies specifically used to address these skills, we are limited in our ability to explain this result. It is possible: (1) that participation in any of these types of youth organizations generally helps young people develop positive coping strategies; (2) young people with better coping skills come to these organizations (i.e., self-select into them); or (3) we might need to do further work on refining the measurement coping in a way that better distinguishes differences.

## Supports and Opportunities

The level of supports and opportunities youth experience during adolescence has been linked to the likelihood that they will achieve good outcomes as young adults (Gambone et al., 2002). This is one of the primary ways that youth settings such as the ones studied here can contribute to the developmental trajectory youth follow and their ultimate ability to thrive as self-sufficient, healthy, contributing members of communities.

Table 4 shows the percentage of youth experiencing optimal or insufficient levels of each of the supports and opportunities for the YLDI agencies classified as identity support (Column I); the YLDI agencies classified as youth organizing agencies (Column II); and the traditional youth development agencies (Column III). We found significant differences in the experiences of youth across the three types of agencies for most of the supports and opportunities measured.

In general, greater percentages of youth in the YLDI agencies than in the traditional youth development agencies report experiencing optimal levels of the supports and opportunities. Only with regard to safety are youth's experiences similar across all types of agencies. Beyond this general trend, however, we noted some differences in the experience of youth depending on the type of YLDI site in which they participated, as well as differences when comparing the YLDI and traditional youth development agencies.

TABLE 4. Youths' Experience of Supports and Opportunities by Agency Type

| | I. Identity Support YLDI Agencies (145) | | II. Youth Organizing YLDI Agencies (65) | | III. General Youth Development Comparison Agencies (257) | | |
|---|---|---|---|---|---|---|---|
| | Insufficient | Optimal | Insufficient | Optimal | Insufficient | Optimal | |
| **Supportive Relationships Overall** | **6%** | **70%** | **6%** | **71%** | **18%** | **52%** | *** |
| Guidance | 6% | 81% | 6% | 82% | 22% | 62% | *** |
| Emotional Support | 7% | 83% | 6% | 88% | 14% | 73% | ** |
| Practical Support | 8% | 77% | 6% | 77% | 22% | 56% | *** |
| Adults' Knowledge of Youth | 43% | 52% | 22% | 68% | 38% | 60% | *** |
| Peer Knowledge of Youth | 26% | 72% | 18% | 78% | 32% | 68% | ns |
| **Safety Overall** | **0%** | **38%** | **0%** | **31%** | **0%** | **29%** | **ns** |
| Physical Safety | 0% | 48% | 0% | 38% | 0% | 45% | ns |
| Emotional Safety | 0% | 61% | 0% | 57% | 0% | 45% | * |
| **Youth Involvement Overall** | **41%** | **4%** | **17%** | **26%** | **41%** | **7%** | *** |
| Decision Making | 32% | 4% | 2% | 31% | 31% | 10% | *** |
| Youth Leadership | 62% | 3% | 23% | 26% | 54% | 4% | *** |
| Belonging | 17% | 43% | 15% | 54% | 27% | 28% | *** |
| **Skill Building Overall** | **30%** | **43%** | **34%** | **26%** | **38%** | **26%** | ** |
| Interesting | 23% | 50% | 25% | 40% | 23% | 27% | *** |
| Growth & Progress | 6% | 50% | 0% | 51% | 17% | 28% | *** |
| Challenging | 11% | 52% | 11% | 38% | 24% | 32% | *** |
| **Community Involvement Overall** | **12%** | **35%** | **3%** | **58%** | **16%** | **24%** | *** |
| Chance to Give Back | 31% | 48% | 14% | 69% | 23% | 49% | ** |
| Knowledge of Community | 16% | 23% | 3% | 72% | 37% | 29% | *** |

***Significant differences between groups at .001
**Significant differences between groups at .01
*Significant differences between groups at .05

*Supportive Relationships.* The YLDI agencies–*youth organizing* and *identity support*–are very similar with regard to the extent they provide youth with supportive relationships overall. In both types of agencies, 70 percent of youth report experiencing consistently supportive relationships (Column I and II). More than 80 percent of youth in both types of agencies receive optimal levels of guidance and emotional support from the adults in these organizations and nearly as many (77%) receive an optimal level of practical support. These results are significantly higher than in the comparison agencies where just over half of youth (52%) report experiencing relationships that are consistently supportive overall (Column III); and significantly fewer youth in these agencies consistently receive guidance, emotional support or practical support from adults.

Qualitative data for YLDI agencies indicate that supportive relationships within these agencies were tied to (1) the types of youth workers and adult volunteers recruited by the agency and (2) the unique qualities of the organizational contexts within these agencies. First, both youth organizing and identity support agencies were successful at recruiting young adults from the community who shared youths' experiences, interests, and backgrounds. In identity support agencies, adults shared the racial, ethnic, cultural, or sexual identity of youth, and could relate to their experiences of marginalization. In youth organizing agencies, youth and adults shared a dedication to various social justice issues and causes. In each case, these similarities helped facilitate positive communication and relationships between adults and youth.

Second, youth organizing and identity support agencies had unique organizational contexts that facilitated relationships. The small size of youth organizing agencies, with small youth adult ratios, created increased opportunities for supportive relationships. Further, youth and adults within youth organizing agencies were engaged in cooperative action, rather than a traditional service delivery model, and this too helped foster respectful and non-hierarchal youth adult relationships. Identity support agencies, on the other hand, placed an explicit and ongoing focus on introducing healthy adult role models into youths' lives. The organizational emphasis on the centrality of relationships in youths' lives translated into the highlighted survey results.

*Safety.* Overall, no differences appear in the proportion of youth who consistently feel safe at these organizations; only about one-third feel both physically and emotionally safe (overall safety). However, with regard to emotional safety, there are significant differences across these organizations; a higher percentage of youth in identity support agencies report consistently experiencing emotional safety compared with those in the traditional youth development agencies.

Qualitative data collected in the YLDI agencies provide a potential explanation for the higher levels of emotional safety in identity support agencies. The organizations that provide identity support activities have a direct focus on the extent to which youth feel emotionally safe (i.e., through the diligent use of communication ground rules and support groups)–which might result in higher proportions of youth deriving this type of benefit from participation.

*Youth Involvement.* As is true for most youth serving agencies, all of the organizations in this study are less successful providing youth with optimal opportunities for meaningful youth involvement than with other developmental experiences. However, greater proportions of youth in the youth organizing agencies report consistently receiving opportunities for meaningful involvement: about one-fourth (26%) of youth in these agencies compared with less than ten percent of youth in either identity support or the traditional youth development agencies.

About one-third (31%) of youth in the youth organizing agencies consistently have opportunities for decision-making, compared with only four percent in identity support agencies and ten percent in traditional youth development agencies. With respect to leadership, about one-fourth of youth in youth organizing agencies report having these types of opportunities compared with less than five percent in other organizations. Similar proportions of youth (about half) in the youth organizing and identity support agencies report a strong sense of belonging compared with only about one-fourth of youth in the traditional youth development agencies.

Qualitative data for YLDI sites suggest that youth leadership is tied to the way youth organizing agencies are structured. Youth organizing groups were more likely to have formal staff and leadership positions for youth than were identity-support or traditional youth development agencies. Formal roles for youth within the agency appear to have translated directly into increased decision-making and leadership roles. Further, youth organizing agencies work closely with a small, core set of youth to train them to lead their larger membership. This intensive focus on a smaller cohort creates more opportunities for leadership within the organization and more time for adults to work one-on-one with youth leaders so that they can succeed in those roles.

*Skill Building.* Overall, higher proportions of youth in the identity support agencies experience optimal levels of skill building compared with youth in either the youth organizing or traditional youth development agencies. However, identity support and youth organizing agencies look similar on each of the dimensions of skill building. (Although a higher percentage of youth in the identity support agencies report that the activities are interesting and challenging than those in youth organizing agencies, the differences are not statistically significant.)

Compared with the traditional youth development agencies, higher proportions of youth in both types of YLDI agency consistently report that their activities are interesting and provide opportunities for growth and progress. And a higher percentage of youth in the identity support agencies find their activities challenging compared with youth in the comparison agencies.

Our qualitative analyses suggest skill building dimensions, such as whether youth feel "interested" and "challenged" by their work, can be difficult to measure with older youth populations. YLDI interviews reveal that youth within youth organizing agencies, for instance, were not consistently interested by some of the daily, routine tasks of organizing (i.e., envelope stuffing, community surveys), and yet are engaged and interested in the overall work of the agency. A finer grained analysis is necessary to tease out youths' perceptions of specific activities or tasks within an agency from their overall skill development.

*Community Involvement.* Youth in the youth organizing agencies clearly have the most opportunity for community involvement. Higher proportions of youth in these agencies consistently experience opportunities to give back to their community and report greater knowledge of their communities compared with youth in both the identity support and traditional agencies. The latter two types of organizations are similar in terms of youths' opportunities to give back to and gain knowledge of their communities.

The community involvement results reflect the structured community focus of the youth organizing agencies, as well as the personal relevance of the issues that youth were addressing. Unlike traditional community service programs, where youth might engage in small and disconnected projects designed to help others, youth organizing agencies worked in a coordinated and strategic effort to reach tangible and personally relevant changes in policy or resource allocation.

## DISCUSSION

Providing any adolescent with the type of environment and experiences that enrich development requires intentionality. Doing so for youth who may be socially and/or politically disenfranchised is often thought to be particularly challenging. At the same time, as the field of voluntary youth organizations matures, there is greater learning about, and recognition of the critical role participation in these organizations play in the outcomes of many youth. The purpose of this paper was to explore whether, and to what extent, civic engagement organizations provide youth with developmental supports–as well as nurture activism. We also sought to explore whether the types of civic activism activities that have youth in leadership roles would be associated with more developmental growth in three key areas.

The paper examined whether civic activism provides an avenue for youth to become active participants in institutions and decisions that affect their lives, while at the same time creating quality opportunities for marginalized and diverse youth to develop holistically. The findings here suggest that civic engagement can fuel both the general development of youth, as well as the development of a sense of social agency–especially as the field learns more about effective practices. The findings also suggest that there are significant differences between types of youth organizations in their achievement of developmental outcomes such as civic activism and identity, and in supports and opportunities such as supportive relationships, youth leadership, decision making, and community involvement. Qualitative data suggest that deliberate approaches to staffing and youth-led decision-making structures can influence the quality of participation and level of outcomes youth experience.

These findings offer some important lessons and insights about promoting youth leadership and involving youth in community that can be instructive for *all* youth development organizations. Promoting high quality youth leadership and community involvement experiences takes well-trained staff, time, and resources. First, staff of the youth organizing and identity support agencies approach their work with older adolescents with much deliberation. They have thought through key issues such as power imbalances between adults and youth, what roles youth can and should play in their organizations and community, the skills and knowledge that staff need, and the skills and supports that youth need to be effective leaders.

Secondly, processes led by youth tend to take more time in order to accommodate and respond to the learning curve youth need. Organizations that seek to support increased youth involvement in decision making need to assess if they are *willing* and *able* to slow down their processes so that youth can play an authentic role. Meaningful community involvement, especially for disaffected youth, also takes time and attention. We found that *if* provided with a structure and framework for identifying challenges in their communities, developing a community change agenda, and engaging in direct action, youth will show the interest and enthusiasm to become more authentically involved in their communities.

Third, we found that clear, focused approaches to promoting youth leadership and community involvement can require more resources. Many of the youth organizing and identity support agencies were specific and targeted in who and how many youth they wanted to reach, primarily due to the background characteristics and the contexts where these youth live. This allowed them to develop a population-specific program curriculum and to develop close, stable, mentoring relationships with youth throughout their leadership and organizing skill training and activism work. In the case of youth organizing groups, this meant a low staff to youth ratio, which allowed staff to work intensely with a relatively small cohort of youth. Since the intentional and deliberate provision of this type of experience appears to be associated with greater levels of developmental supports and outcomes, the youth field needs to begin to explore how more of these experiences can be provided more broadly to youth.

Finally, this paper presents a comparative analysis based on a small convenience sample. There would be great value in further studies that address questions of attribution and causation. For example, are the youth drawn to community youth development organizations fundamentally different than those who attend traditional youth development groups? What extraneous factors influence participation in community youth development organizations? In addition, longitudinal studies of individual level outcomes would help answer at least three important questions: (1) Does receiving higher levels of supports and opportunities in a program setting result in higher levels of civic engagement outcomes? (2) Are youth more likely to attain positive developmental outcomes the longer they stay in a program? (3) Can these developmental outcomes be directly related to desired long-term outcomes including economic self-sufficiency, healthy family and social relationships, and civic involvement? Information from these studies will provide critical knowledge to better design youth programs and train practitioners to enable youth to be effective change leaders in their communities.

# REFERENCES

Camino, L., & Shepherd, Z. (October 2002). From periphery to center: Pathways for youth civic engagement in the day-to-day life of communities. *Applied Developmental Science*, *6*(4), 213-220.

Connell, J. P., Gambone, M. A., & Smith, T.J. (2000). Youth development in community settings: Challenges to our field and our approach. In *Youth development: Issues, challenges and directions* (pp. 281-300). Philadelphia: Public/Private Ventures.

Gambone, M. A., Klem, A., & Connell, J. (2002). *Finding out what matters for youth: Testing key links in a community action framework for youth development.* Philadelphia: Youth Development Strategies, Inc., and Institute for Research and Reform in Education.

Hughes, D., & Curnan, S. (2002). Towards shared prosperity: Change-making in the CYD movement. *Community Youth Development Journal*, *3*, 25-33.

Irby, M., Ferber, T., & Pittman K. with Tolman, J. & Yohalem, N. (2001). *Youth action: Youth contributing to communities, communities supporting youth.* Community & Youth Development Series, Vol. 6. Takoma Park, MD: The Forum for Youth Investment, International Youth Foundation.

Kahne, J., Honig, M.I., & McLaughlin, M.W. (2002). The civic components of community youth development. *CYD Anthology*.

Larson, R., & Hansen, D. (2004). The development of strategic thinking: Learning to impact human systems in a youth activism program. *Human Development 272*, 1-23.

Lewis-Charp, H., Yu, H.C., Soukamneuth, S., & Lacoe, J. (2003). *Extending the reach of youth development through civic activism: Outcomes of the youth leadership development initiative.* Social Policy Research Associates.

Michelsen, E., Zaff, J. F., & Hair, E.C. (2002). *Civic engagement programs and youth development: A synthesis.* Washington, DC: Child Trends.

Mohamed, I., & Wheeler, W. (2001). *Broadening the bounds of youth development: Youth as engaged citizens.* A Joint Publication of the Ford Foundation and The Innovation Center for Community and Youth Development.

Sherrod, L. (2000). The development of citizenship in today's youth. A special issue of the *Journal of Applied Developmental Science*.

Sullivan, L. (1997). Hip-Hop nation: The underdeveloped social capital of Black urban America. *National Civic Review*, *86*(3), 235-244.

Torney-Purtra, J. (1999). Conference Consensus Paper: Creating citizenship: Youth development for free and democratic society. Retrieved March 2004, from http://www.Stanford.edu/group/adolescent center.ctr/Conference/consens1.html

Torney-Purta, J., Lehmann, R., Oswald, H. & Schultz, W. (2001). *Citizenship and education in twenty-eight countries: Civic knowledge at age fourteen.* Amsterdam: International Association for the Evaluation of Educational Achievement.

# Index

# BOOK ORDER FORM!

Order a copy of this book with this form or online at:
http://www.HaworthPress.com/store/product.asp?sku= 5861

## Youth Participation and Community Change

___ in softbound at $21.95 ISBN-13: 978-0-7890-3292-8 / ISBN-10: 0-7890-3292-9.
___ in hardbound at $39.95 ISBN-13: 978-0-7890-3291-1 / ISBN-10: 0-7890-3291-0.

COST OF BOOKS _____

POSTAGE & HANDLING _____
US: $4.00 for first book & $1.50
for each additional book
Outside US: $5.00 for first book
& $2.00 for each additional book.

SUBTOTAL _____
In Canada: add 7% GST. _____

STATE TAX _____
CA, IL, IN, MN, NJ, NY, OH, PA & SD residents
please add appropriate local sales tax.

FINAL TOTAL _____
If paying in Canadian funds, convert
using the current exchange rate,
UNESCO coupons welcome.

❏ BILL ME LATER:
Bill-me option is good on US/Canada/
Mexico orders only; not good to jobbers,
wholesalers, or subscription agencies.

❏ Signature _____

❏ Payment Enclosed: $_____

❏ PLEASE CHARGE TO MY CREDIT CARD:
❏ Visa ❏ MasterCard ❏ AmEx ❏ Discover
❏ Diner's Club ❏ Eurocard ❏ JCB.

Account #_____

Exp Date _____

Signature _____
(Prices in US dollars and subject to change without notice.)

### PLEASE PRINT ALL INFORMATION OR ATTACH YOUR BUSINESS CARD

Name

Address

City                    State/Province                    Zip/Postal Code

Country

Tel                                    Fax

E-Mail

May we use your e-mail address for confirmations and other types of information? ❏ Yes ❏ No We appreciate receiving
your e-mail address. Haworth would like to e-mail special discount offers to you, as a preferred customer.
**We will never share, rent, or exchange your e-mail address. We regard such actions as an invasion of your privacy.**

Order from your **local bookstore** or directly from
**The Haworth Press, Inc.** 10 Alice Street, Binghamton, New York 13904-1580 • USA
Call our toll-free number (1-800-429-6784) / Outside US/Canada: (607) 722-5857
Fax: 1-800-895-0582 / Outside US/Canada: (607) 771-0012
E-mail your order to us: orders@HaworthPress.com

**For orders outside US and Canada,** you may wish to order through your local
sales representative, distributor, or bookseller.
For information, see http://HaworthPress.com/distributors

(Discounts are available for individual orders in US and Canada only, not booksellers/distributors.)

**Please photocopy this form for your personal use.**
www.HaworthPress.com

BOF06